Hypertension Essentials

Current Concepts of Cause and Control

Hypertension Essentials

Current Concepts of Cause and Control

THEODORE L. GOODFRIEND, M.D.

Professor of Internal Medicine and Pharmacology
University of Wisconsin School of Medicine
and
Associate Chief of Staff for Research
William S. Middleton Memorial Veterans Hospital
Madison, Wisconsin

1983

G&S

GRUNE & STRATTON

A Subsidiary of Harcourt Brace Jovanovich, Publishers

New York London
Paris San Diego San Francisco São Paulo Sydney Tokyo Toronto

Library of Congress Cataloging in Publication Data

Goodfriend, Theodore L.
Hypertension essentials.

Bibliography: p.
Includes index.
1. Hypertension. 2. Hypertension--Chemotherapy.
3. Hypotensive agents. I. Title. [DNLM: 1. Hypertension.
2. Hypertension--Drug therapy. 3. Antihypertensive agents.
WG 340 H996503]
RC685.H8G65 1983 616.1'32 82-11604
ISBN 0-8089-1534-7 (Cloth)
0-8089-1583-5 (Paper)

Grune & Stratton, Inc.
111 Fifth Avenue
New York, New York 10003

Distributed in the United Kingdom by
Academic Press Inc. (London) Ltd.
24/28 Oval Road, London NW 1

Library of Congress Catalog Number 82-11604
International Standard Book Number 0-8089-1534-7 (Cloth)
0-8089-1583-5 (Paper)

Printed in the United States of America

To my parents, Tess and David,
for the preparation.

To my children, David and Michael,
for the expectation.

To my wife, Mary Lou,
for the inspiration.

Contents

***This chapter was written in collaboration with Dr. Enid F. Gilbert, Professor of Pathology, University of Wisconsin School of Medicine, Madison, Wisconsin.**

Preface

It has always been second nature for physicians to pay attention to blood pressure. It is a sign of life, one of the "vital signs." At first, pressure was palpated at the pulse, then measured more precisely using the sphygmomanometer. Without hurting the patient in the slightest, a clinician can measure intravascular pressure with a precision of about 2%! This remains one of the most accurate measurements in medicine.

When statistics accumulated by life insurance companies proved that blood pressure elevation shortened life, attention to blood pressure escalated. Now it is a topic of conversation for everyone from schoolchildren to their grandparents. The following book is dedicated to keeping its readers ahead of those who read the lay press and to improving the care of hypertensives, whatever they read.

The goal of the medical approach to hypertension is very simple: *lower the pressure!* High pressure damages blood vessels and the heart, regardless of the underlying cause. Lowering pressure improves longevity, regardless of the (ethical) methods used to lower it.

It is fortunate that the medical goal is so simple and the choice of tools so broad, because it is impossible to understand the cause of hypertension in most cases, and it is very difficult to tailor therapy to individual patients. We should bear in mind that despite our ability to *treat* virtually all hypertension, we can *cure* almost none of it.

In the course of trying to understand hypertension, we have learned a great deal about the normal control of blood pressure. In the course of trying to find the perfect treatment, we have devised a large variety of reasonably effective drugs and techniques. This book (like all of medical education) will pay attention to those aspects of hypertension that are well understood: normal regulation of blood pressure, the rare diseases in which hypertension results from known causes, the damage caused by elevated pressure, and the known aspects of treatment modalities. Of necessity, we will omit what is *unknown*: the cause of hypertension in 90% of cases, the precise mechanism by which most drugs lower blood pressure, the way to cure hypertension so treatment can be stopped, and the way to prevent hypertension so that books like this will be superfluous.

Acknowledgments

This book comes from one pen guided by many minds. Dr. Harold Itskovitz first interested the author in hypertension and has continued to introduce new concepts into our understanding of this condition. The welcome proferred by Drs. F. Merlin Bumpus, Philip Khairallah, and Harriet Dustan gave the author his first insight into the potential intellectual challenges and rewards in the study of hypertension. The Cleveland Clinic has remained a deep and accessible wellspring of new information about hypertension, dating from its long inspiration by Dr. Irvine Page.

The author is especially indebted to his students, who not only endured his evolution as a teacher and writer, but who also contributed specific criticisms and additions to the text. John Bohn, Brian Templeton, and Arthur Schuna reviewed the entire manuscript and made many valuable comments. Specific suggestions were also offered by Joellen Altschaefl, Todd Anderson, Kathy Cox, Barb Hansen, Ann Holmquist, Chris Huiras, Randall Kieser, Gary Kubalak, Mark McDermott, Joyce Miller, Todd Patton, Mary Quarto, David Rapkin, John Rosebush, Matthew Samore, David Scherwinsky, Frank Sheski, Tom Sinksy, Linnea Smith, Sister Shirley Stingle, and Mike Vrabec.

The chapter on pathology in this volume was written in collaboration with Professor Enid Gilbert of the University of Wisconsin School of Medicine.

The author was blessed by the patient and expert assistance of his secretary, Mrs. Beverly Birdsall, and by the creative artistry of Mr. Robert Zelm, the graphic artist at the Madison V.A. Hospital.

1

Control of Arterial Blood Pressure in Normal Humans

Introduction

This volume begins with a discussion of normal arterial pressure, its function, mechanism, and regulation. We know much more about normal than pathological aspects of blood pressure. As we will see toward the end of this book, treatment of *high* blood pressure is directed at eroding the *normal* supports of blood pressure. Until the cause of common hypertension is understood, normal mechanisms are all that can be attacked.

Functions of Arterial Blood Pressure

One function of arterial blood pressure is to move the blood around the body, exposing tissues to the blood's ability to carry gases. This requires very little pressure. The gases diffuse from red cell to tissue cell without help from hydrostatic pressure in the blood. However, the huge bed of capillaries and arterioles has an intrinsic resistance to flow, the blood is somewhat viscous, and it has to move fast enough to bring oxygenated red cells to respiring cells. We can assume this requires pressure equal to about 5 millimeters of mercury (mm Hg) (1 mm Hg = 1 torr).

A second function is to squeeze fluid out of the blood, exposing cells to nongaseous nutrients such as glucose and amino acids. This requires hydrostatic pressure to overcome the colloid osmotic pressure of the plasma. Colloid osmotic pressure is about 25 mm Hg.

A third function is to overcome gravity (behold, the giraffe!) and opposing pressures, such as intracranial pressure and resistance generated by contracting muscles. Gravity alone requires a pressure of 30 mm Hg in a tall human.

A fourth function is to enable regulation of blood flow under varying demands, such as exercise. In other words, to have the capacity to regulate flow, some variable resistance must be present. This is the property of arterioles with muscular walls; while constricted, they offer resistance. This necessitates hydrostatic pressure to allow *some* flow past the resistance, if not the tissue beyond would die. This requires 10 mm Hg.

The *minimum* arterial pressure required for life depends on posture (upright or horizontal), intracranial pressure, and tissue resistance. A patient on an operating table, with widely dilated vessels, and enough circulating blood volume to fill them, can survive with an arterial pressure of 50–70 mm Hg.

Pressures higher than the minimum requirement are attenuated between the heart and the tissues by arteriolar constriction. This protects the tissues from the mechanical trauma of high blood pressure and prevents one-way transudation of excess plasma fluids from capillaries.

Note that this list, and virtually all of the book to follow, is concerned only with *arterial* pressure. Venous pressure is a study in itself; it participates in arterial pressure regulation by propelling blood into the heart and is subject to some of the same influences as arterial pressure (vasconstrictor hormones, fluid intake, etc.). It will not be considered in detail in this volume.

Definitions and Principles

Systolic arterial pressure is the peak pressure achieved during cardiac contraction. *Diastolic* pressure is the lowest pressure during cardiac relaxation. *Mean* pressure is the mean of the integrated pressure during the entire cycle; it can be estimated as the diastolic pressure plus one-third the difference between diastolic and systolic. (*Pulse* pressure is the difference between systolic and diastolic.) (Remember, diastolic pressure is especially important for coronary perfusion.)

Pressure is measured in major arteries, such as the brachial, which are proximal to the resistance vessels (the arterioles). Flow through capillaries is measured in other, indirect ways, such as skin temperature, urinary output, cardiac function, level of consciousness, and plasma lactate. Therefore, ''blood pressure'' as we know it is a measurement one-step-removed from the most important *function* of the pressure, perfusion of the tissues. Thus, a patient could have ''normal'' blood pressure, but not be perfusing the tissues because of vasoconstriction between the large vessels and the capillaries. Or at a very ''low'' pressure, perfusion could be adequate, because the blood vessels were widely vasodilated.

Although pressure in the larger arteries is *not* the final determinant of flow-through capillaries it *is* the major determinant of vascular pathology. It is primarily because of pathology, not perfusion, that we study arterial blood pressure. Furthermore, it is in the major vessels—of the same size as those in which pressure is measured—that high blood pressure does its greatest harm. Atherosclerosis of primary and secondary branches from the aorta is the greatest health danger facing modern industrial man; it is accelerated most prominently by hypertension, and it is the pressure in those vessels that we customarily measure.

Evidence That Pressure Is Regulated

Each person, normal or not, has a characteristic pressure which fluctuates with exercise, sleep, etc. After these fluctuations, the pressure returns to its characteristic mean level. This return to a prior level is achieved by the pressure-regulating mechanisms discussed below.

Regulation of Pressure

Coarse Adjustments

Pressure in a *dynamic,* moving fluid is determined by the nature of the fluid, the pump, and the resistance in the pipes. This is expressed mathematically by the physiological version of the well-known voltage equation (Ohm's law):

$$\text{BP} = \text{Cardiac Output} \times \text{Peripheral Resistance}$$

The nature of the fluid in the system affects pressure only when its *viscosity* changes. This rarely happens in humans, except in cases of polycythemia, hyperglobulinemia, or macroglobulinemia. (Otherwise, cardiac output and peripheral resistance tell the whole story.)

A second way of looking at pressure is to imagine the cardiovascular system as *static,* like a balloon. Then, pressure is directly proportional to intravascular fluid volume and inversely proportional to capacity:

$$\text{Pressure} \sim \frac{\text{Volume}}{\text{Capacity}}$$

In thinking about *hypertension,* it is simpler to talk about the static model and concern oneself with blood volume and vascular capacity. In thinking about

TABLE I

Control Loops That Affect Arterial Blood Pressure Listed According to the Sensor

Sensor	*Stimulus*	*Pathway and effectors*
1. Carotid sinus and aortic arch baroreceptors (high-pressure baroreceptors)	Pressure change in arterial system	Nerve impulses to brain, then changes in cholinergic and adrenergic regulation of heart, vessels, adrenals and kidneys
2. Right atrium and other central volume receptors (low-pressure baroreceptors)	Blood volume (venous return to the heart)	Same as above
3. Carotid and aortic bodies	Oxygen (pO_2), CO_2, pH of plasma	Same as above
4. Macula densa	Sodium in urine	Renin–angiotensin–aldosterone
5. Juxtaglomerular apparatus	Pressure across glomerulus in kidney	Renin–angiotensin–aldosterone
6. Osmoreceptors	Osmolality of plasma	Vasopressin (ADH)
7. Hypothalamus	pO_2, pCO_2, pH of plasma	Nerves to vessels, heart, and kidneys
8. CNS	Environmental stress, excitement, cerebral ischemia	Catecholamines, nerve impulses
9. Renal filtering apparatus	Mean arterial pressure	"Pressure–dialysis," the extrusion of plasma fluid into urine through glomerulus
10. Renal medulla	?	Prostaglandins and other depressor lipids
11. Parenchymnal cells of peripheral organs	Blood flow	Kinins, adenosine, CO_2, lactate, etc. (These result in "autoregulation" of *flow* to match metabolic *demands*)
12. Individual vessels	Pressure	Direct effects of pressure to dilate vessels ("stress–relaxation)

shock, it is simpler to talk about the dynamic model and concern oneself with cardiac output and peripheral resistance.

These two ways of looking at pressure (dynamic and static) can be combined, because cardiac output is dependent on the relative volume of intravascular fluid. The amount of blood whipping around the system and entering the right atrium determines the force and volume of the heart's output. More blood volume causes more cardiac output (and higher arterial pressure). More will be said about this later.

Fine Adjustments

There are many regulatory systems participating in control of blood pressure. Most of them were discovered during short-term experiments on dogs. The majority are probably important only for short-term regulation (e.g., during bursts of exercise and changes of position). However, only the regulators that set long-term pressure are important in the slow vascular damage caused by chronic hypertension. The major unknown in blood pressure regulation is the definition of the factor(s) that determine long-term pressure settings in humans.

All control loops can be described by: their stimuli (or "signals"); sensors; effectors; pathways; and feedback characteristics (e.g., "gain"). The accompanying tables look at the control loops in three ways: sensors (Table I), effector organs (Table II), and chemical mediators (Table II).

TABLE II

Organs and Chemical Mediators Affecting Blood Pressure

Organs effecting changes in pressure (the efferent limbs of control loops). Each organ can participate in more than one control system.

1. Heart
2. Arterioles and veins
3. Kidney
4. Adrenal cortex
5. Adrenal medulla and sympathetic nerves
6. Brain

Chemical Mediators of pressure control. This list helps you think of lowering BP by chemical antagonists. Each of these may act on more than one organ and participate in more than one control loop.

1. Angiotensin
2. Aldosterone and other steroids } The "Three A's" (items 1–3)
3. "Adrenaline" (and norepinephrine)
4. Prostaglandins and kinins
5. Unknown mediators of local changes in flow
6. Vasopressin (?)

Advantages and Disadvantages in the Complex Pressure-Regulating System

Advantages to this system include the following:

1. Cooperation of many components theoretically permits rapid and certain responses to emergencies, plus fine-tuning capabilities.
2. "Fail-safe" and "backup" systems enable ablation of entire components without total loss of control (e.g., in adrenalectomy, nephrectomy, or heart transplants).
3. Complexity allows local changes to supersede systemic ones in vital organs, such as heart and kidney.

Flaws inherent in the complex regulating system include the following:

1. The independence of sensors from each other is a potential danger. For example, renal or cerebral ischemia can over drive the system and cause vascular disease elsewhere, because local conditions near one sensor may not be true of the body as a whole.
2. The system fails to sense the capacity of effectors to perform. For example, the kidneys can drive the heart to exhaustion in demanding arterial pressure for glomerular filtration.
3. The existing set of regulatory loops fails to sense *total* fluid volume, focusing only on intravascular volume. Large accumulations of fluid, such as ascites and edema, are ignored.
4. The system fails to sense the *absolute* level of pressure. Thus, hypertensive patients resist a return to normal pressure. Their sensors are "re-set" to the abnormal pressure.
5. The multiple loops fail to avoid "snowballing" or "piling on" of compensatory changes. For example, in renal hypertension, catecholamines are overproduced as are renin, angiotensin, and aldosterone.
6. Some sensors, such as the baroreceptors, fail to monitor *flow* through tissues adequately. (However, sensors in the brain and kidney, and chemoreceptors do look at flow as well as pressure.)
7. Multiple components make it difficult to *treat* elevations of pressure (see later chapters).

Orchestration of the Components of Regulation

Each regulatory component has its own characteristics: the pressure domain it guards, the duration of its effects, and its efficiency.

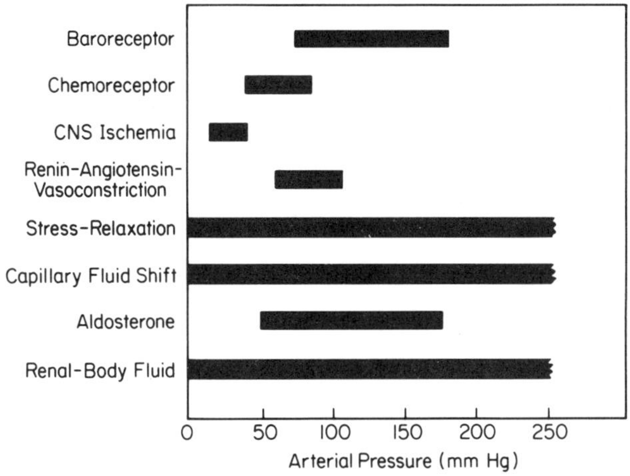

Fig. 1. Levels of arterial blood pressure that are buffered by various pressure-regulating systems (after Guyton). Not all systems operate at all pressures. Some have fairly narrow domains.

Individual components have separate jurisdictions based on the *ranges of pressures* that activate them and turn them off again (see Fig. 1). At average or high pressures, the baroreceptors are in play; at low pressures, the brain is fighting to restore pressure; and at all levels, the kidneys and vessels buffer pressure changes.

Individual components have their own *time* characteristics (lag, duration, fatigue) (see Fig. 2). Baroreceptors are short acting whereas kidney, brain, and vessels are long acting.

Individual components have their own *efficiency* or "gain," (i.e., how *well* they restore pressure to normal; see Fig. 2).

Figures 1 and 2 shown how Guyton ranks and classifies the pressure regulators. Note how short-lived the effects of the baroreceptors are. They quickly "fatigue" or "adapt." Thus, it is unlikely that baroreceptor abnormalities cause *lifelong* hypertension. By contrast, abnormalities of vessels causing them to fail to stretch or relax with increasing pressure could affect pressure throughout life. The kidneys will be considered separately in the next section.

Kidneys as the Dominant Pressure Regulator

By Guyton's analysis, the *kidneys* are the dominant influence on *long-term* pressure regulation, although not on short-term adjustments. His reasoning goes something like this:

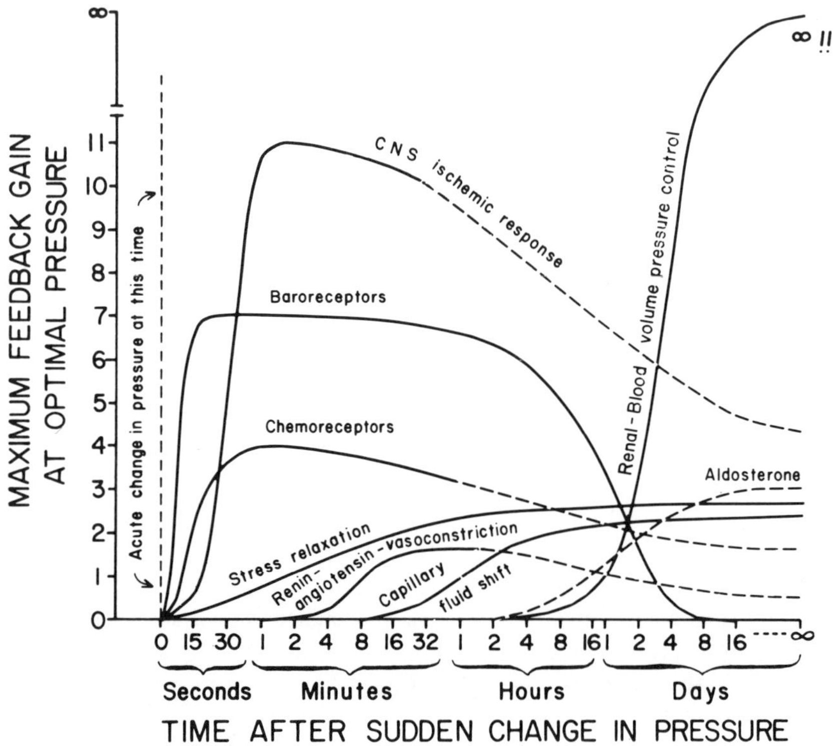

Fig. 2. Duration of effects of various blood pressure-regulating systems after a stimulus that perturbs them and the efficacy (''gain'') of each system to restore pressure to the original level (after Guyton). Note how different the regulatory systems are with respect to speed of onset, duration of effectiveness, and degree to which they restore pressure to control levels.

1. Pressure is the resultant of cardiac output and peripheral resistance. The kidneys can *change* blood pressure as follows:
   a. Fluid retention by the kidneys causes increased venous blood returned to the heart.
   b. More blood returning to the heart increases cardiac output.
   c. Increased cardiac output causes many tissues to ''autoregulate'' (to maintain constant flow) by constricting arterioles. Autoregulation of flow is a prominent characteristic of brain and kidney, and possibly of other organs. This ''total body autoregulation'' causes a rise in total peripheral resistance.
   d. Thus, fluid retention by the kidneys causes an increase in both the cardiac output *and* peripheral resistance. The net effect is a rise in

blood pressure. (Of course, increased fluid *excretion* would cause a *fall* in pressure by the reverse sequence.)

2. The kidneys *respond* to blood pressure as follows:
   a. The kidneys excrete sodium and fluid in proportion to arterial pressure. (This is a general fact that supersedes the effects of aldosterone, antidiuretic hormone, etc.) At higher pressures, more fluid is excreted, and at lower pressures, less fluid is excreted. This is the Central Dogma of the Guyton formulation (see Fig. 3).
   b. Thus, pressure determines net fluid output; and, as described above, fluid output determines pressure. These two parameters are tightly linked. The tightness of their linkage is a measure of how much this particular regulatory system determines pressure. By Guyton's analysis the linkage is perfect, since there is clearly no loss or gain in extracellular volume through the course of time as

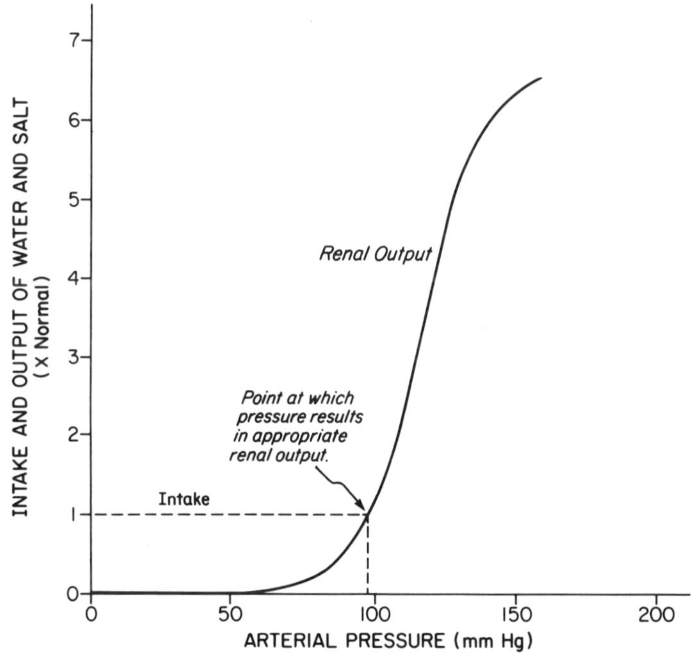

Fig. 3. Relationship between arterial blood pressure and fluid excretion by the kidneys. Higher pressure results in greater fluid output. The dotted line shows how much fluid is excreted at the indicated pressure. In reverse, this relationship describes the effects of fluid intake on arterial pressure. Increased fluid in the cardiovascular tree results in higher arterial pressure (after Guyton).

the intake of sodium and water fluctuates. A little extra intake must raise pressure slightly and cause the kidneys to excrete a little extra urine. This perfect balance reflects a feedback control loop of "infinite gain." This extremely high gain means that of all the pressure-regulating loops, the pressure-kidney loop must be the dominant one (see Fig. 2).

3. One implication of this formulation involves the relationship between oral salt and water intake and pressure. (Note: Unless indicated otherwise the term "salt" is intended to mean *sodium* chloride. Because sodium is the major cation of the plasma, sodium salts are those in which intake affects plasma volume.) All the salt and water ingested must be excreted by the kidneys. Increased intake requires increased excretion, and increased excretion demands increased pressure. So according to Guyton, an increased blood pressure *must* result from either increased salt intake or decreased renal capacity to excrete salt at

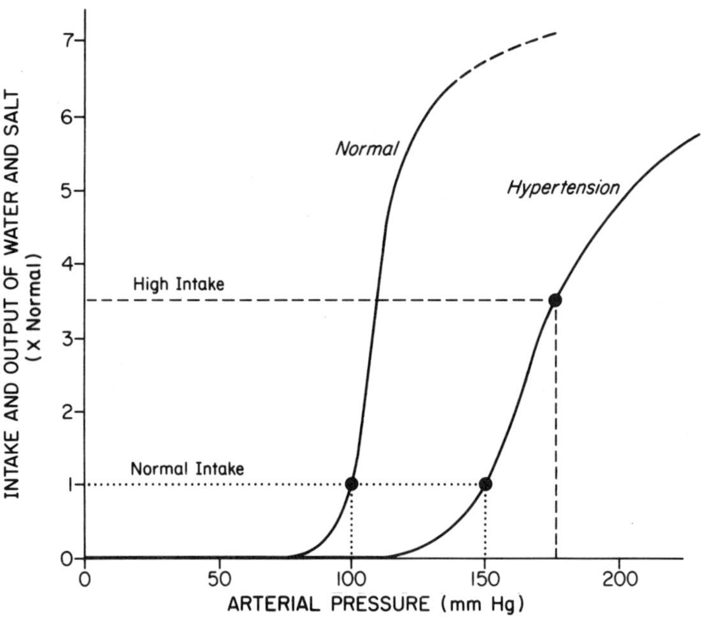

Fig. 4. Relationship between arterial pressure and fluid excretion by the kidneys in normal and abnormal patients and the effects of increased salt (and water) intake on aıterial pressure in normals and abnormals. Blood pressure can be increased by changing the relationship between pressure and excretion (i.e., by changing the kidney), or by increasing the requirement for fluid excretion (i.e., by increasing salt and water intake).

a given pressure. A hypertensive patient, for Guyton, is a person with excessive salt intake, or subtly inept kidneys, who constantly requires increased pressure to excrete salt. This formulation would explain the key role of both salt and the kidneys in hypertension (depicted graphically in Fig. 4).

4. The final component of Guyton's formulation is "autoregulation." This term signifies the ability of organs to adjust their own blood flow, despite fluctuations of pressure. It may seem logical that organs be able to open up their arteries when pressure falls. (That ability saves our brains from ischemia every morning when we get out of bed.) The converse also takes place: *when arterial pressure rises, many arterioles constrict to keep flow constant.* Apparently, our organs try to prevent over-perfusion as well as under-perfusion. (This makes sense in the kidney, where over-perfusion could lead to fluid excretion, but it makes less apparent sense in other organs whose function might be profitably increased, like the brain!) According to Guyton, increased cardiac output leads to widespread autoregulation and increased total peripheral resistance. A hypertensive patient, by this analysis, may start out with excessive cardiac output and peripheral blood flow, but autoregulation will convert the patient to one with excessive peripheral resistance.

There is some experimental evidence that supports Guyton:

1. In hypertensive rats, transplantation of the kidneys causes the recipient rat to assume the pressures of the donor (i.e., pressure follows the kidneys).
2. In humans with reduced renal function, pressure is often determined by sodium and water intake. These are the "volume-dependent" hypertensives. Their pressures are clearly dependent on the kidneys' ability to *excrete* sodium. If that is limited, the intake of sodium becomes a major determinant of pressure.

There is also some evidence against Guyton:

1. Patients with essential hypertension have *reduced* plasma volume. How could they be driving their pressures up by a renal defect causing fluid *retention?* Guyton responds by maintaining that these patients are in the advanced stage of his formulation. At that stage, autoregulation has taken over, and peripheral resistance is sustaining the high arterial pressure.
2. Many drugs appear to lower pressure without affecting the kidneys. Guyton argues that subtle changes in the kidneys that will change

pressure cannot be detected by current methods, and that drugs acting primarily on the nervous system may actually have subtle effects on the kidneys.

3. Some of the classical causes of hypertension, such as pheochromocytoma, show no apparent structural abnormalities in the kidneys. Guyton replies that these are instances of a constant chemical influence on the kidneys, rather than a structural or functional defect in the kidneys. We could detect the renal change if we had appropriate tools.

The Brain and Nervous System as Dominant Pressure Regulators

Ever since it was observed that excitement or stress raised blood pressure, it has been postulated that the brain is the dominant regulator of pressure. Even the term "hypertension" implies to some people that there is increased emotional "tension" in patients with the disease.

When the pathways carrying impulses from the brain to the heart and vessels were found to flow through the autonomic system—whose transmitters were largely catecholamines—the hypothesis "tension → autonomic pathways → catecholamine release → vasoconstriction and increased cardiac output → hypertension" was constructed.

The earliest drugs that lowered pressure interrupted the postulated pathway by sedating the patients (e.g., bromides and barbiturates). The first successful antihypertensive drugs were blockers of autonomic ganglia. The next good drug was reserpine, which depletes central and peripheral nerve cells of catecholamines. At that point, the hypothesis of a central or autonomic origin for hypertension looked very good.

With the advent of oral diuretics and their success in lowering pressure, attention shifted to the kidney as the dominant pressure regulator. The apogee of this line of thought is the Guyton hypothesis described above.

Newer evidence again points to the brain as the dominant (or "codominant") regulator of the long-term pressure set-point. This evidence includes the following:

1. Even in severely hypertensive patients, pressure drops during sleep.
2. Many of the newest drugs that successfully lower pressure affect the brain (e.g., methyldopa, clonidine, propranolol).
3. Some hormones that raise pressure, such as angiotensin, have dramatic effects when applied directly to localized areas in the brain (hypothalamus and floor of the third ventricle). This suggests that their pressor

effects may be mediated by actions on the brain as well as on peripheral vessels or kidneys.

4. If some areas of the brain are ablated experimentally, hypertension fails to develop when classic pressor manipulations, such as experimental renal artery stenosis, are done. Pressure also fails to develop in genetically inbred hypertensive rats if these critical brain areas are zapped when the animals are young.

A hypertensive patient, according to this school of thought, is someone whose master-control center in the brain is set at too high a level. As a result, all systems under nervous control are driven to maintain the abnormal pressure. What remains unexplained in this hypothesis is the precise nature of the brain pathology that leads to the elevated set-point in the first place.

Guyton's thesis would rebut all this evidence by simply saying that nervous impulses and transmitters exert their ultimate effects on pressure by an intermediate effect on the kidney.

It is well known that *increased intracranial pressure* causes a compensatory rise in arterial blood pressure in order to assure perfusion of the brain. This phenomenon demonstrates the ability of the brain to raise blood pressure, but does not bear on the role of the brain in chronic, essential hypertension, where intracranial pressure is normal.

Vessels as Dominant Pressure Regulators

Since peripheral arterial resistance is one of two ultimate variables by which pressure is regulated (the other being cardiac output), it is natural to attribute high pressure to tight vessels. Furthermore, every hypertensive eventually gets thickened arterial walls. In the late stages of hypertension, patients do have increased total peripheral resistance. Guyton says that the *vessels in the kidneys* may well be the place where abnormal pressure arises. A similar story can be constructed for the role of abnormal *vessels in the brain*. Whether abnormal vessels are CAUSE or EFFECT of hypertension (or BOTH CAUSE AND EFFECT) remains unproved.

Implications of Theories for Genesis and Therapy of Hypertension

Fixed hypertension is the result of either *constant abnormal stimuli*, an *abnormal set-point* of one or more pressure sensors, or *abnormal integration* of the reflexes by the brain or kidney. Diagnosis should begin by searching for abnormal sources of stimuli (chemical mediators) or abnormal integrators (kidneys).

Therapy should be directed, ideally, at removing abnormal pressor stimuli, readjusting pressure sensors, or correcting the "integrator." These goals are currently beyond us, except in a small percentage of patients.

Available therapy is now based on blunting several known *normal* pressor systems at the same time (by using either one drug with many sites of action or more than one drug at the same time). This approach begs the question of which system is abnormal. It is "shot-gun therapy" in the truest sense of the word.

Summary

The best-established facts about pressure regulation are these:

There are multiple regulatory systems affecting blood pressure. Each has its characteristic signal, sensor, and effector pathway. Each also has its own range of pressures to work on, its characteristic strength of response, and its typical duration of effect.

The probable long-term regulators of pressure are kidneys, brain, and peripheral vessels.

Many pathological changes in the kidneys can lead to elevated pressure.

The interaction of the kidneys, sodium, fluid, and blood pressure can be summarized as follows: a drop in arterial pressure leads to retention of salt and water; increased salt and water intake raises arterial pressure unless the kidneys are made to excrete sodium more readily; and any change in renal handling of salt and water affects blood pressure unless intake of salt and water are modified to compensate for the changed kidneys.

The nervous system can raise or lower blood pressure quickly and dramatically, and experimental lesions in the brain can prevent chronic elevations of pressure.

The mechanisms that determine the mean pressure carried through life, whether normal or abnormal, have not been clearly specified.

2 The Renin–Angiotensin–Aldosterone System

Introduction

This chapter describes a complex system that affects blood pressure, blood volume, and serum potassium concentration. The renin–angiotensin–aldosterone system is a favorite subject of examination writers. Until recently, its role in therapy was primarily to foil it. Now, we have drugs that inhibit various parts of this system, so intelligent treatment requires that we understand how it works. It is also a system altered by two of the classic "curable" causes of hypertension, renal artery stenosis and hyperaldosteronism.

Teleology

The renin–angiotensin–aldosterone system regulates blood pressure and sodium excretion on behalf of a vital organ, the kidney, to protect it from reductions in blood flow. It serves the kidney at the expense of other organs that might need blood, such as muscles and viscera.

The renin–angiotensin–aldosterone system is primarily concerned with plasma *volume,* especially the *effectiveness* of plasma volume in perfusing the kidneys. Other hormones, such as insulin, parathormone, and antidiuretic hormone (vasopressin), are involved in regulating the *composition* of plasma, although aldosterone can regulate the concentration of plasma K^+ and H^+. (K^+ and H^+ are excreted in exchange for sodium retained under the influence of aldosterone.)

The osmoreceptors are so adept at holding plasma water concentration constant that the *concentration of sodium* does not change appreciably, no matter how dramatically aldosterone affects its excretion.

Components

Organs involved in synthesis of components are

1. The *juxtaglomerular* (JG) *apparatus* of the kidneys is the site of synthesis of renin.
2. The *liver* is the site of synthesis of renin substrate (angiotensinogen).
3. The *plasma* is the site of angiotensin synthesis.
4. The *lung* is the site of conversion of inactive angiotensin I to active angiotensin II.
5. The *adrenal glomerulosa* (the outer zone of the adrenal cortex) is the site of synthesis of aldosterone.

Renin (pronounced "ree-nin" not "rennin") is an enzyme made first in a "prorenin" (precursor) form, and then activated to renin, which is released into the blood by the JG apparatus. (Some prorenin is found in plasma too. It is especially high in the blood of diabetics and patients with renin-producing tumors.) Renin is *in*activated by the liver.

Renin substrate (angiotensinogen) is a globulin found in the plasma in large amounts (enough to make 1000 times more angiotensin than would be active on most vessels). It is formed in the liver.

Angiotensins are the small polypeptides formed from renin substrate by the enzymatic action of renin. The reactions take place in the plasma in two or three steps:

1. Renin Substrate $\xrightarrow{\text{renin}}$ Angiotensin I (10 amino acids)

2. Angio I $\xrightarrow[\text{enzyme}]{\text{converting}}$ Angiotensin II (8 amino acids)

3. Angio II $\xrightarrow[\text{A}]{\text{angiotensinase}}$ Angiotensin III (7 amino acids)

Angiotensin III is also called des-aspartic^1-A II, because it lacks the aspartic acid in position 1.

Converting Enzyme (angiotensin converting enzyme or "ACE") is localized at endothelial cell membranes, in contact with blood, mostly in the lung. It is poised there to convert angiotensin I in venous blood into angiotenin II in arterial blood. The same enzyme is a vicious kininase, destroying the vasodilator bradykinin. Thus, converting enzyme *creates* a *vasoconstrictor* (angiotensin II), and *destroys* a *vasodilator* (bradykinin).

Angiotensin II constricts blood vessels, primarily the arteries and arterioles. Angiotensins II and III stimulate aldosterone production by the zona glomerulosa of the adrenal cortex.

Aldosterone acts on sites where sodium can be lost, to reduce this loss (kidney, sweat glands, salivary glands, and colon). Consequent to retention of sodium is retention of water (if the antidiuretic hormone system is working) and preservation of the extracellular fluid volume. Extracellular fluid is the stuff from which plasma is made. In the renal tubule where aldosterone acts, sodium reabsorption from the urine is linked to potassium and hydrogen ion excretion into the urine.

There are less well-known effects of the angiotensins that also support the blood pressure and plasma volume: effects on the brain cause stimulation of drinking and release of antidiuretic hormone that result in water retention, effects on the heart result in increased myocardial contractility, effects on nerves and adrenal medulla cause release of catecholamines, and stimulation of CNS pressure centers raises pressure by mobilizing the brain's integrative capacities. There is also some evidence that angiotensins have their own, intrinsic aldosterone-like activity on the kidney, causing sodium retention directly.

Probably, the individual beds of vessels adjust local distribution of blood flow by their variable responsiveness to angiotensin and their capacity to release prostaglandins. This is particularly true in the kidney. It would be self-defeating for angiotensin to shut down the kidneys. When angiotensin is injected into kidneys, vasodilating prostaglandins are released that antagonize angiotensin's vasoconstriction there. (The prostaglandins are destroyed by the lung, so they do not antagonize angiotensin's systemic effects.)

This system is a major supporter of blood pressure *when blood volume is reduced,* when sodium is lost, or when sodium intake is low. One of the best stimuli for turning on the system is hemorrhage; another is diuresis. In normal, sedentary, sodium-loaded Americans, the renin–aldo system is "off," plasma renin levels are low and the system is not active in supporting blood pressure. It can also be turned "on" by upright posture and exercise, by dehydration (e.g., sweating), and by salt restriction. All of these events reduce blood volume and threaten perfusion of the kidneys.

Regulation of Renin Release

The major site of regulation of the renin–angiotensin–aldosterone system is the *JG apparatus* where *renin* is *released.* The other components of the system are all present in excess, e.g., substrate, converting enzyme, angiotensinases, and aldosterone-secreting capacity.

Effective perfusion of kidney is the key regulator in renin release.

1. The JG apparatus senses perfusion of the kidney by two parameters: *pressure in the afferent arteriole and the concentration of sodium chloride in the distal tubular urine.*
2. When effective perfusion is low, so is pressure at the afferent arteriole where the JG cells are located. When perfusion is low, so is glomerular filtration of sodium. Most of the sodium chloride is reabsorbed before it hits the distal tubule whose contents are being "tasted" by the macula densa of the JG apparatus. Apparently, both low pressure and low urinary sodium stimulate renin release.

Sodium chloride depletion alone also causes renin release, even when pressure and perfusion are normal. If very little salt and water are filtered by the glomerulosa, all the salt can be reabsorbed in the proximal tubule, the macula densa will taste little salt at the distal site and the JG cells will release renin in response to this sodium deficiency.

Sympathetic nerves to the kidneys can cause renin release. There are reflexes ending in these nerves that start with receptors in the *right atrium.* These are called "low-pressure baroreceptors," because atrial pressure is low. They "sense" right atrial filling. When the volume of circulating blood is low, venous return is relatively slow, the right atrium is small, the reflex is triggered, and sympathetic nerves to the JG apparatus are stimulated. There are probably other stimuli that can activate these nerves, especially excitement. The sympathetic nerves release catecholamines, and the receptor in the juxtaglomerular cells that triggers renin release is a β_1 adrenergic receptor.

When effective circulation *to the kidney* is restored to normal after a volume-depleting event such as hemorrhage, renin release is turned off.

There are direct *chemical* stimuli and inhibitors affecting renin release by cellular mechanisms inside the JG apparatus. These chemicals include *angiotensins,* which reduce renin release by direct feedback inhibition; *catecholamines* and *prostaglandins,* which stimulate renin release directly; and *potassium,* high levels of which turn *off* renin release. In brief, catecholamines and prostaglandins stimulate renin release, angiotensins and potassium inhibit it.

The multiplicity of factors that can affect renin release result in a well-

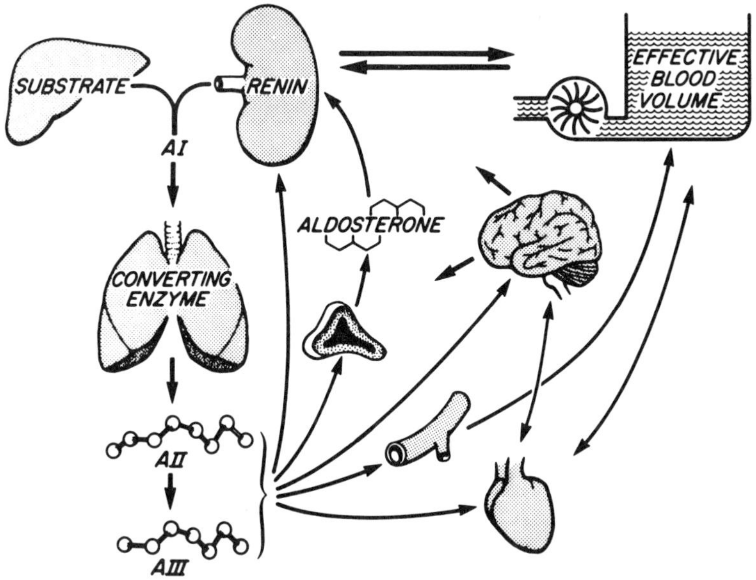

Fig. 1. A schematic diagram of the renin–angiotensin–aldosterone system, showing the formation of angiotensins (on the left) and the organs they affect (on the right). The final feedback regulator of the system is "effective blood volume." It is depicted here as a volume of liquid that can do useful work (on a turbine, in this diagram). Effective blood volume regulates release of renin, and is affected in turn by all aspects of the system.

buffered system. It is almost impossible to shut off renin release completely. Figure 1 summarizes some interactions of the renin–angiotensin–aldosterone system.

Regulation of Other Components of the Renin–Angiotensin–Aldosterone System

Renin substrate (angiotensinogen) levels in the blood are increased during pregnancy, and following estrogen administration (e.g., oral contraception). This is a direct effect of these hormones on the synthesis of renin substrate by the liver. However, the release of renin from the kidney falls when renin substrate in plasma rises. This is the result of feedback inhibition of renin release by the extra angiotensin formed from excess substrate. Thus, when estrogens are administered, the renin substrate level rises, but renin enzyme concentration falls. The net effect is only a *slightly* elevated renin activity in plasma. (Note the use of two terms, "concentration" and "activity," describing plasma renin. Renin concentration is only one determinant of renin activity; others include the concentration of substrate and pH.)

Aldosterone secretion can be stimulated directly by increased blood levels of angiotensin, potassium, or ACTH. There is some dispute about the precise role of ACTH in aldosterone secretion. ACTH probably *supports* aldosterone synthesis, but is not *necessary* for it. Hypopituitary patients with no ACTH have normal *basal* aldosterone secretion, and their zona glomerulosa is intact while the rest of the adrenal atrophies. (However, the zona glomerulosa does not respond well to sodium depletion in patients with abnormal pituitary glands, even though renin levels rise. Something in the pituitary gland must sensitize the adrenal glomerulosa to angiotensin; it may or may not be ACTH.)

Pathophysiology with *High* Renin Levels

Renin, angiotensin, and aldosterone levels are *increased* in the blood in the following situations, all of which are characterized by reduced perfusion of the kidneys and reduced venous return to the right atrium:

1. Hemorrhage
2. Diuresis
3. Salt depletion (in low sodium diets, etc.)
4. Dehydration
5. Adrenal insufficiency (renin and angiotenin levels may be up, but of course, that of *aldosterone is down* because the adrenal itself is sick)
6. Upright posture for 1–2 hr (doubles the plasma renin concentration)
7. Nephrotic syndrome or hypoalbuminemia
8. Cirrhosis with ascites
9. Heart failure

(Note that in 7, 8, and 9 total body sodium and water may be up, but the blood flow to the kidneys is down, because the fluid is largely collected in tissue spaces such as the peritoneal cavity. In a condition like ascites, there is not only a good deal of fluid in a nonvascular space, but that fluid may obstruct venous return further by pressure on the abdominal veins.)

The renin–angiotensin–aldosterone system is also stimulated in the following conditions *without* depleted blood volume:

1. *Stenosis of the renal artery* or diseases of small arteries of the kidney can reduce blood flow to the JG apparatus even though perfusion pressure at the aorta is normal and the sodium supply is high. This

causes a paradoxically high level of renin release and can lead to *renovascular hypertension*. In that case, pressure in the rest of the body is raised above normal in an attempt by the kidney to achieve normal pressure at the glomeruli.

2. There are *renin-secreting tumors* of the kidney that can cause confusing syndromes. These are usually variants of Wilms' tumors. Recently, a case of pancreatic carcinoma producing renin was reported. The clinical picture in patients with renin-producing tumors includes hypertension, thirst, and low serum potassium.
3. "*Bartter's Syndrome*" is a rare, familial condition characterized by the following:
    a. High plasma renin and angiotensin levels, high aldosterone levels, low plasma potassium levels, but *normal blood pressure*.
    b. Apparently, the vessels in patients with Bartter's Syndrome do not respond to angiotensin, but the adrenal glomerulosa zone does.
    c. In the kidney, there is *JG hyperplasia*.
    d. Because the aldosterone level is high, sodium is retained and *potassium lost*.
    e. Blood pressure is paradoxically normal in the face of high renin levels.
    f. This syndrome probably originates with a renal defect in *chloride* reabsorption leading to *chloride and potassium loss* that somehow stimulates *prostaglandin release*. The prostaglandins then stimulate renin release, but they also block angiotensin's pressor effects on vessels. Prostaglandins do not block angiotensin's effects on the adrenal gland. The high angiotensin level then stimulates the adrenal glomerulosa, causing increased aldosterone production. Aldosterone's effects on the kidneys aggravate the original potassium loss even further.
    g. The syndrome is partially reversed by drugs that block prostaglandin synthesis (e.g., aspirin and indomethacin). Without the stimulus of prostaglandins, renin release falls, so the aldosterone level returns to normal. In addition to aspirin-like drugs, these patients need potassium supplements to replenish their severely depleted body stores, and to compensate for the continuing loss of potassium caused by the basic tubular defect.
4. In a variety of renal diseases, glomerular perfusion is reduced, or JG cells are damaged, and renin release is either stimulated or renin leaks out of the damaged JG cells. These conditions include malignant hypertension and some cases of "end-stage renal disease."

Pathophysiology with *Low* Renin Levels

When sodium intake is high, when fluids are over-infused, or when the adrenal makes too much aldosterone or other mineralocorticoids, the body fluid compartments are full and the renin level is very low in the blood. The most quoted example is a tumor of the adrenal glomerulosa that makes excessive aldosterone called *aldosteronoma* or *Conn's tumor*.

In some cases of diabetes and in some patients with renal disease, renin secretion from the kidney can be inappropriately low. These patients also have low levels of aldosterone and tend to develop high potassium levels. This condition is called *Hyporeninemic Hypoaldosteronism*.

Some dysautonomias (diseases of the autonomic nervous system such as Shy-Drager Syndrome) have low renin secretion. This results in a failure of renin release in response to upright posture and contributes to the *postural hypotension* these patients suffer.

High potassium levels lower renin release. This is a direct effect of potassium on the JG cells. There is also the direct effect of high potassium levels on the adrenal to increase aldosterone secretion. This seems paradoxical at first, but actually, makes sense. In a case of high K^+ the action of aldosterone would be useful, causing loss of K^+ into the urine. However, there is no need for vasoconstriction, so it would be inappropriate to call for the aldosterone by releasing renin. Instead, the high K^+ acts directly on the adrenal gland to release aldosterone and directly on the JG cells to turn off renin release.

Some patients with hypertension have low renin levels for unexplained reason(s) (Low Renin Essential Hypertension). This will be discussed again in a subsequent chapter.

Pharmacology

Renin release is *stimulated* by the following chemicals:

1. Catecholamines. This is a direct effect on the JG cells that have adrenergic receptors of the β_1 type that usually respond to catecholamines released by the renal nerves or in the circulating blood.
2. Diuretics. Some act directly on JG cells as well as indirectly by fluid loss.
3. Vasodilators (e.g., hydralazine, diazoxide, and prostaglandins). They lower blood pressure and stimulate JG pressure sensors. Prostaglandins also act directly on JG cells.
4. Inhibitors of angiotensin or its formation. These prevent feedback inhibition by angiotensin (see below).

Renin release is partially *inhibited* by the following chemicals:

1. Antisympathetic drugs (e.g., propranolol, methyldopa, prazosin, and clonidine). These drugs reduce renin release caused by nervous stimuli, but do not completely block the effects of low blood pressure or low sodium concentrations in the tubular urine.
2. Inhibitors of prostaglandin synthesis (like aspirin and indomethacin). Remember that prostaglandins (especially prostacyclin-PGI_2) stimulate renin release by direct effects on JG cells. Drugs like aspirin reduce renin release, but do not eliminate it.

Angiotensin Converting Enzyme (ACE) is blocked by a drug called "captopril" (Capoten®). The drug may also cause a *rise* in *bradykinin* concentration, since converting enzyme normally destroys bradykinin. The unexpected success of this drug in lowering pressure in patients with *normal* plasma renin activity (in addition to its expected success in patients with *high* plasma renin activity) suggests that the renin system is more important in typical hypertensives than was previously appreciated.

Angiotensin can be blocked at its receptors by peptides that are competitive inhibitors, such as saralasin (Sarenin®), (sarcosine^1, alanine^8-angiotensin). This must be given iv, since it is a peptide that would be digested in the gut if taken by mouth. Its best use is in diagnosing renin-dependent forms of hypertension.

Angiotensin's action to cause vasoconstriction can be reversed by *vasodilators* such as nitroprusside or prostaglandins. This is an effect of the vasodilators on muscle in the vessel, not on angiotensin or its receptors.

Aldosterone can be blocked at its receptors by spironolactone (Aldactone®), a competitive inhibitor.

Aldosterone's effects on sodium can be overcome by *diuretics* that poison the sodium pump(s) in renal tubule cells. This is not a specific antialdosterone effect.

Renin substrate synthesis is increased by estrogens, such as the oral contraceptives.

Diagnostic Uses of Renin

Instead of measuring the absolute levels of various components, laboratories measure *plasma renin activity,* (PRA). This enzyme activity is a resultant of the concentration of enzyme and the concentration of substrate.

PRA is high or low in the conditions listed on pp. 20–22 and summarized in Table I.

Because it is such a physiologically variable parameter, peripheral PRA is not very useful in diagnosis of diseases—too many other things in addition to

TABLE I

Changes in Plasma Renin Activity (PRA)[a]

Increased	*Decreased*
1. Hemorrhage	1. *Aldosterone-secreting tumor*
2. Diuresis	2. *Adrenal hyperplasia*
3. Salt depletion	3. Excessive salt ingestion
4. Dehydration	4. *Hyporeninemic hypoaldosteronism*
5. Adrenal insufficiency	5. Dysautonomia
6. Upright posture	6. *Low-renin essential hypertension*
7. Nephrotic syndrome	7. High potassium levels (hyperkalemia)
8. Cirrhosis with ascites	8. Therapy with antiautonomic drugs
9. Heart failure	9. Nonsteroidal antiinflammatory drugs
10. *Renin-secreting tumor*	
11. *Bartter's Syndrome*	
12. Malignant hypertension	
13. Vasodilator therapy	
14. Therapy with converting enzyme blockers	
15. Exercise or stress	
16. Pregnancy or estrogen therapy	
17. *Renal artery stenosis* (raises PRA in blood from affected kidney)	
18. *Volume-independent hypertension of renal failure* (see Chapter 4)	

[a] Italicized conditions are those in which the measurement of renin can be of clinical value.

the disease can change PRA. However, it has specific value in the diseases italicized in Table I.

Renal vein bloods are sampled for renin levels when renal artery stenosis is suspected. In that disease, renal venous renin levels are *very* useful, whereas the peripheral (arm vein) venous renin level is less so.

Summary

The renin–angiotensin–aldosterone system is very well understood and can be blocked by new drugs like captopril. By constricting vessels, retaining sodium, and other effects the system helps support normal pressure in people deprived of salt and in emergencies that threaten blood volume. It is the key mediator of abnormal blood pressure in unilateral, renal artery stenosis and some other renal diseases, and it probably helps to maintain pressure in many other kinds of hypertension.

3 Selected Aspects of the Autonomic Nervous System

Introduction

The autonomic nervous system affects so much physiology that a full description would fill a huge volume. This chapter outlines the system briefly and emphasizes those parts that impinge directly on arterial blood pressure. In the chapters on autonomic inhibitory drugs, the side effects described there will comprise a summary of the other functions of this system, since no drug has yet appeared that affects only the cardiovascular domain of autonomia.

Major Divisions of Autonomia

The autonomic nervous system can be divided biochemically into cholinergic and adrenergic parts, and anatomically into parasympathetic and sympathetic parts. The cholinergic (parasympathetic) system employs acetyl choline as its final effector molecule, whereas the adrenergic (sympathetic) system employs the catecholamines epinephrine, norepinephrine, and dopamine. In anatomic terms, the cholinergic system employs the vagus nerve to carry most of its visceral impulses, whereas the adrenergic system employs the sympathetic nerves and the adrenal medulla.

It is still useful to think of the cholinergic (parasympathetic, vagal) system as the director of "vegetative" functions. A good prototype of cholinergic dominance is a cow in a meadow—eating, excreting, salivating, and snoozing, with slow pulse and low blood pressure. By contrast, the adrenergic (sympathetic) system designed for "emergencies" is embodied by a gazelle fleeing a lion on the Serengetti Plain—heart vigorously pumping, blood shunted to the muscles under high pressure, all metabolism geared to producing glucose, with the digestive tract temporarily at rest (although we humans might do some precipitous excreting under similar circumstances).

Most organs are supplied by both adrenergic and cholinergic nerves, usually exerting opposite effects. A good example of this duality is the vessels supplying skeletal muscles. These vessels are affected by both adrenergic and cholinergic nerves. The state of the blood vessels at any one time is the result of the opposing systems.

Major Subdivisions of the Adrenal Nervous System: α, β, and Dopaminergic Postsynaptic Receptors

The adrenergic (sympathetic) system executes three types of functions: α adrenergic, β adrenergic and dopaminergic. α-Adrenergic functions are best stimulated by norepinephrine, β functions by epinephrine, and dopaminergic by dopamine. Norepinephrine has considerable β activity even though it is the classical α agonist. Specificity within the sympathetic system is accentuated by specialization of receptors. Although the chemical effectors can cross-react, the receptors in target organs are more specific.

The typical α-adrenergic function is contraction of vascular smooth muscle in most arteries. Typical β adrenergic functions are increased rate and force of the heartbeat and dilation of the bronchi and vessels to muscles. The typical peripheral dopaminergic function is dilation of the arteries in the kidneys.

Further Subdivisions of the Adrenergic Nervous System

Classical adrenergic receptors are *postsynaptic,* residing on the effector cells, such as vascular smooth muscle, and triggering its activity. One of the newest wrinkles in sympathetic nervous system physiology is the description of *presynaptic* receptors. They sit on the nearside of the synapse. Released catecholamines swing back on their cell of origin and affect further synthesis by interacting with presynaptic receptors.

α-Adrenergic functions, mediated classically by norepinephrine, are subdivided into α_1 and α_2 by virtue of specific receptors. α_1 Receptors trigger the classical response of vasoconstriction. They are postsynaptic, residing on the far side of the cleft that separates nerve fiber from effector organs such as vascular smooth muscle.

α_2 Receptors are in two locations, presynaptic and central. *Presynaptic* α_2 receptors mediate *a reduction in catecholamine production.* In this way, they exert a negative effect on α adrenergic activity. They are part of a negative feedback loop initiated by release of norepinephrine into the synapse. Part of the released norepinephrine triggers α_1 receptors on the far side of the cleft causing vasoconstriction and part triggers α_2 receptors on the cell that released the hormone, turning off its further synthesis. α_2 Receptors located on presynaptic neurones have a negative effect on blood pressure, reducing catecholamine production.

α_2 Receptors in the brain are also "negative" in their effect on blood pressure, mediating a reduction of sympathetic nerve impulses leaving the brain. We are not sure how this is achieved in cellular terms.

β-Adrenergic functions, mediated classically by epinephrine, are subdivided into β_1 and β_2 by virtue of specific receptors. β_1 Receptors are found in the heart, and mediate the classic increase in rate and force of cardiac contraction that typifies adrenergic activity.

β_2 Receptors reside in bronchial smooth muscle, in vessels to skeletal muscle, and in muscle and liver cells. In smooth muscle, β_2 receptors mediate the relaxation that dilates bronchi and vessels. In liver and muscle, they trigger the biochemistry that converts glycogen to glucose.

Both β_1 and β_2 receptors are found in the central nervous system; their functions are not known precisely, but they clearly play a major role in orchestrating sympathetic nerve traffic to the periphery.

The best-characterized β receptors are postsynaptic, on effector cells. In addition, there is good evidence for *presynaptic* β *receptors*. They apparently *increase norepinephrine synthesis* (opposite to the inhibitory presynaptic α_2's).

Summary

A summary of autonomic subdivisions and their effects is found in Table I. A schematic representation of a synapse between an adrenergic nerve and a vascular smooth muscle fiber is presented in Fig. 1.

It is *impossible* to divide the autonomic nervous system into easy-to-remember divisions with respect to blood pressure. α Receptors were classically

TABLE I

Autonomic Nervous System Effects[a]

Organ	Adrenergic (sympathetic)				Cholinergic (parasympathetic)
	α_1	α_2	β_1	β_2	
Heart	—	—	Increase strength and rate of contraction	—	Slow rate of contraction
Arteries to muscles	Constrict	Reduce synthesis of NE	—	Dilate	Dilate
Arteries to skin	Constrict	Reduce synthesis of NE	—	—	Dilate
Kidneys	Constrict[b] arteries	—	Release renin	—	—
Cerebral blood pressure-regulating centers	?	Reduce pressure impulses	Stimulate pressor impulses	?	?
Bronchi	—	—	—	Dilate	Constrict
Gut	Close	Decrease motility	—	Decrease motility	Increase motility and secretion, relax sphincters
Fat cells	—	Inhibit lipolysis	Stimulate lipolysis	—	—
Platelets	—	?	Stimulate aggregation	—	—

[a] — Indicates no effect. ? Indicates presence of receptor but uncertain function.
[b] Dopamine causes vasodilation in kidneys, probably by interacting with specific dopaminergic receptors.

thought of as pressure raisers. Postsynaptic α_1 receptors responding to norepinephrine can still be considered classic pressor receptors. But the newly discovered α_2 receptors that turn off norepinephrine synthesis (presynaptic α_2's, and those α_2's that turn off sympathetic outflow from the brain are clearly *depressor* receptors. The same paradoxes exist in beta-ville.

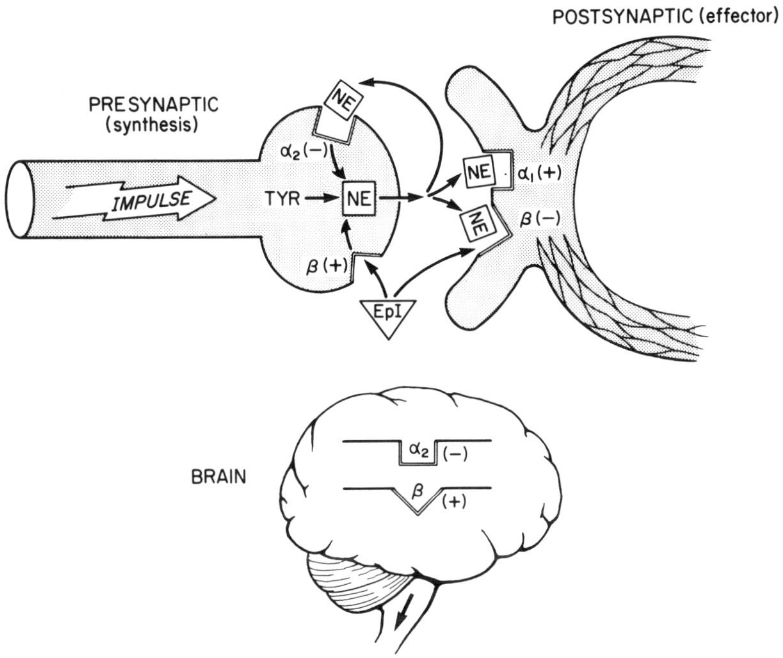

Fig. 1. Diagram of a typical adrenergic synapse. The afferent nerve synthesizes norepinephrine. The effector is a vascular smooth muscle cell. The blood pressure effects of synaptic norepinephrine and circulating epinephrine interacting with α NE or β EpI , NE receptors on either side of the synapse (and in two prototypic areas of the brain) are indicated by + or − signs.

4 Well-Understood ("Curable") Causes of Hypertension: I. Renal Diseases

Introduction

The kidneys are extremely important in regulating blood pressure over the long term, and diseases of the kidneys are frequently accompanied by hypertension. There are at least three ways the kidneys can raise blood pressure: by retaining sodium and water, and thus affecting blood volume; by secreting renin; and by failing to secrete pressure-lowering hormones such as prostaglandins and kinins.

Renal Failure

Although kidneys can fail in a variety of ways (e.g., fail to excrete acid, fail to excrete potassium), when renal failure causes *hypertension* it is because the kidneys *fail to excrete sodium*. Pressure in this condition is dramatically modified by sodium intake. This is clearly an example of Guyton's hypothesis in action. This type of hypertension is called ''volume-dependent hypertension.'' (The volume referred to is blood volume.) These patients have pressures that respond dramatically to changes in blood volume induced by hemodialysis on an artificial kidney.

In some cases of renal failure, salt restriction or volume contraction (even when it is achieved by hemodialysis on the artificial kidney) fails to lower pressure. In such cases the hypertension is ''volume-independent.'' These patients frequently have a renal disease that results in *renin secretion*.

"Renoprival" Hypertension (A Concept, Not a Disease Entity)

Renoprival refers to the hypertension accompanying complete loss of both kidneys. In such a case hypertension could be caused by excessive sodium retention and blood volume expansion (but it could *not* possibly be caused by renin!)

Since the kidneys secrete pressure-*lowering* substances, such as prostaglandins and kinins, it is possible that renoprival hypertension is caused or worsened by *de*ficiency of these *de*pressors.

To review: prostaglandins are products of the metabolism of arachidonic acid. The vasodilating prostaglandins are PGI_2 (''prostacyclin'') and PGE's. (Vasoconstricting ones are PGF's and thromboxanes.)

The kinins are small polypeptides (e.g., bradykinin and kallidin) that are cleaved from a plasma globulin (''kininogen'') by enzymes called ''kallikrein.'' The kidneys are rich in kallikrein, some of which is excreted in the urine and some of which acts on plasma kininogen to release kinins into the blood. The kinins are extremely potent vasodilators (with other properties that roughly resemble histamine). Kinins are extremely rapidly destroyed by enzymes, including angiotensin-converting enzyme (ACE).

The role played by prostaglandins and kinins in hypertension is completely unknown. Because these substances are so potent, and because they affect blood vessels, it is tempting to attribute a powerful influence to them. However, there is very little evidence to support this role. For example, aspirin-like drugs inhibit prostaglandin synthesis, but have very little effect on blood pressure.

Renal Diseases Causing Hypertension

Acute

Acute renal diseases, such as glomerulonephritis, are frequently accompanied by *sodium retention* and edema, and renin levels that are either absolutely high or ''inappropriately high.''

Chronic

Chronic (parenchymal) renal diseases include such conditions as chronic glomerulonephritis, chronic pyelonephritis, or nephrosclerosis (atherosclerosis of renal vessels).

1. Under these conditions, the mechanism of hypertension is not clear, because there may be no demonstrable failure of sodium excretion, a normal blood urea nitrogen (BUN) level and creatinine, and no apparent elevation of renin in the plasma. Could this type of disease be another example of the Guyton hypothesis, but with a defect in sodium excretion that is too subtle to be detected by current methods? Whatever the mechanism, chronic parenchymal renal diseases are probably the most common renal causes of hypertension.
2. Hypertension, from whatever cause, *results* in nephrosclerosis. This is a specific example of the acceleration of atherosclerosis that results from hypertension. Therefore, it is almost impossible to tell how much kidney disease is *cause* and how much is *effect* in most chronic cases of hypertension.
3. If chronic renal disease accompanied by hypertension is *unilateral,* it is unlikely that the renal disease is the *result* of hypertension. Hypertension should accelerate vascular disease everywhere. In such cases it would be worth considering surgical removal of the diseased kidney to relieve the hypertension.
4. Almost every renal disease (except salt-losing nephropathy) is accompanied by, or aggravates, preexisting hypertension. The list is long and includes: urinary tract obstruction, polycystic disease, emboli and infarcts, hematomas, and intrinsic and metastatic tumors. Although these conditions may be associated with hypertension, the mechanism of the pressure rise they cause is uncertain.

Malignant Hypertension

Whatever initiates hypertension, it can, when it gets out of hand, affect the kidneys, damaging them in an apparently mechanical way. It seems that the bounding pressure simply beats the kidneys to death. This causes excessive release of renin from the damaged JG cells; and that starts a vicious cycle (high pressure → high renin → higher pressure, etc.). Malignant hypertension is almost always accompanied by high plasma renin activity. It will be discussed again in the context of hypertensive emergencies.

Renin-Secreting Tumors (Hemangiopericytomas or Wilm's Tumors)

Most common in children, renin-secreting tumors cause hypertension by releasing huge quantities of renin into the blood.

Renal Artery Stenosis (Responsible for 2–5% of All Hypertension)

The lesions of renal artery stenosis can affect small or large vessels, in one or both kidneys. To cause hypertension (i.e., to be "physiologically significant"), the lesion must have a precise effect on blood flow to the kidney. Too little stenosis and there is no renin release, too much stenosis and there is death of the kidney (and a dead kidney soon releases no renin). The usual guideline for physiological significance is 90% occlusion. However, collaterals can muddy the picture and perfuse glomeruli behind a total obstruction, resulting in renin release.

There are many possible pathological causes of stenosis. In younger females *fibromuscular dysplasia* is common. In older patients *atherosclerosis* is most common. In addition, renal circulation can be impaired by emboli, extrinsic pressure from tumors, "kinking" of the vessel after transplantation, or the many types of microscopic "horrors" arteries are prone to.

When stenosis affects only *one* kidney or only part of the total renal mass, the mechanism of hypertension is almost certainly excess release of *renin*, followed by generation of angiotensin and expression of its effects on vessels, adrenal, etc.

When stenosis is bilateral or affects most of the vessels to the glomeruli, the mechanism of hypertension is probably a *combination* of *renin release* and *inadequate excretion of sodium*.

In both unilateral and bilateral stenosis, the level of peripheral plasma renin is increased early in the disease, but returns to normal late in the disease. Apparently, excess renin–angiotensin–aldosterone results in fluid retention, which tends to shut off renin even while the arterial constriction persists. However, even in the late stages, with renin near normal, repair of the stenosis can cure the hypertension. This suggests that the *near-normal* renin level is still *too high*.

Diagnosis

The clinical *history* is helpful in raising suspicion of renal artery stenosis if there has been flank pain (indicating a renal infarct), sudden onset of hypertension, sudden worsening of hypertension, or if there is an absence of any family history of hypertension. Occurrence of severe hypertension in females under 40 with no family history is suspicious of renal artery stenosis. One useful clue to the existence of *bilateral* renovascular hypertension is an increase of BUN or creatinine when pressure is lowered with drugs. (In unilateral disease, the normal kidney can excrete all nitrogenous wastes.)

The *physical exam* is helpful only if there is a renal artery *bruit audible in the abdomen* or over the back at the costovertebral angles. One should listen below the ribs anteriorly for a continuous or back-and-forth high-pitched ''whoosh.'' About 40% of patients with renal artery stenosis have a bruit with a diastolic component. Only about 1% of people without stenosis have a bruit extending into diastole. (The more common whoosh that occurs in systole alone is simply a sign of aortic atherosclerosis.)

The easiest radiographic screening test for renal artery stenosis is the *intravenous pyelogram* (IVP), with iv administration of dye and ''rapid sequence'' films thereafter (the so-called hypertensive IVP). However, this will detect only about 80% of all patients with renal artery stenosis. The test also has about 10% *false positives,* suggesting renal artery stenosis when none exists. There are five changes to look for in the IVP:

1. One kidney smaller than the other by 1.5 cm
2. Slow uptake of dye
3. Increased concentration of dye
4. Slow washout of dye
5. Notching of ureter by collateral vessels from below

The newest twist to the IVP is one in which the contrast is enhanced by a computer. This is called ''digital subtraction arteriography.'' The computer subtracts the preinjection image from images made as dye is injected intravenously. By this technique, an *intravenous* injection can be used to visualize the *arteries* as dye recirculates from vein-to-heart-to-arteries.

The most specific test for renal artery stenosis is *arteriography,* with injection of dye into the aorta and/or the renal arteries themselves. It is difficult to judge whether the observed stenosis is exerting a pathological effect, i.e., causing renin release. Two bits of circumstantial evidence of ''functionally significant stenosis'' would be *poststenotic dilation* of the vessel and the presence of *collaterals*. Both imply that the stenosis is causing problems downstream and is probably stimulating release of renin.

''*Renograms*'' are nuclear medicine procedures in which IVP dye is labeled with radioiodine, and recorded by geiger counters instead of X-ray film. It is like an IVP without the pictorial detail. In renograms, as with IVP, one looks for delayed appearance of the dye in the stenosed kidney and for delayed washout of the dye from the kidney. This test uses a trace amount of the radiolabeled IVP dye, so it is especially useful in patients who are allergic to the dye. It is a poor test for renal hypertension caused by stenosis of small, segmental arteries.

The best prognostic test is the measurement of *renal vein renins* (renin in the venous blood from both normal and abnormal kidneys). If the ratio of levels in the blood from the affected to the normal side is greater than 1.5 : 1.0, not only is there likely to be *a physiologically significant stenosis,* but the results of surgery are likely to be good (93% of patients with an abnormal renin ratio have good surgical results). This test demonstrates that the stenosis is triggering renin release and contributing to hypertension. Therefore, relief of the stenosis will almost certainly remove one of the contributors to hypertension. If one or both kidneys *also* have severe parenchymal disease (e.g., nephrosclerosis), surgery will not help, and hypertension may persist after surgery. Usually, whatever hypertension persists after surgery is easier to treat with drugs than it was before surgery.

Renal renin ratios are less useful when arterial disease is *bilateral.* In that situation, renin levels only point to the worst kidney, they do not dictate whether or not bilateral surgery will be needed. The IVP and renogram are also poor detectors of stenosis occurring on *both* sides. The arteriogram is the best test for those cases. See the following paragraph for a pharmacological test useful in bilateral stenosis.

The newest test for renovascular hypertension involves the use of *angiotensin antagonists* (e.g., saralasin) or *converting-enzyme blockers* (e.g., captopril). A dramatic drop in pressure when these drugs are given will reveal those patients whose pressure is being supported by the renin–angiotensin system whether the underlying cause is unilateral renal disease, bilateral renal disease, tumor, etc. However, even normals or patients with essential hypertension get pressure support from this system at times (e.g., sodium restriction). Therefore, there are likely to be a good many false-positive tests. Furthermore, the test will not identify those patients with a *treatable* lesion, as opposed to those with such things as diffuse renal disease. However, such a test could be a good screening device under proper control.

The goals of diagnosis are to detect those patients with hypertension who have a *treatable* renal vascular lesion and to make an estimate of the value of proposed surgery. Arteriograms would *find* lesions, but would not indicate whether the stenosis was causing hypertension, nor accurately predict the results of surgery. Renal vein renins are good *prognosticators,* but cannot localize lesions precisely or evaluate the feasibility of repair. (Neither is a good screening test for a large population.)

A *diagnostic scheme* for patients suspected of having renal artery stenosis is as follows:

1. History, physical examination, urinalysis and serum BUN or creatinine, and a rapid-sequence IVP can all be done without admitting patients to the hospital. If the patient has a bruit with a diastolic component and an abnormal IVP, he has a 90% chance of having renal artery stenosis.
2. Admit patients with suspicious findings and perform simultaneous arteriograms and sampling of renal vein bloods for measurement of renin. These tests can be done at the same time by a radiologist skilled in the use of vascular catheters.

Treatment

Drugs vs Surgery

Debate rages between advocates of surgery and advocates of drugs. Both modalities are becoming more effective. Surgery is preferred when the lesion is relatively easy to repair and the patient is young. Surgery is more likely to be successful when renal vein renin from the affected side is 1.5 times as high as the other side; it is less likely to be successful when patients have disseminated atherosclerosis with angina, diabetes, extensive bilateral renal disease with elevated creatinine, or are relatively old (over 55).

Drugs are indicated in old or diabetic patients who have atherosclerosis everywhere, patients who will not tolerate surgery, or patients with lesions that are hard to repair (e.g., multiple, small stenoses). It is reasonable to try drugs first in patients where the risks of surgery are relatively high and to operate if drugs fail.

The availability of captopril and saralasin makes it possible to use drugs as a diagnostic probe. A dramatic response to one of these blockers of the renin–angiotensin system suggests not only that drugs could be used in chronic treatment, but also that correction of the stenosis will lead to a reduction of pressure.

Goals

There are two goals of treatment: lowering of blood pressure and preservation of renal function. With stenosis present, the "normal" kidney is bombarded with high pressures and develops nephrosclerosis, whereas the abnormal kidney (the stenotic one) is *protected* from high pressure by its own stenosis! If surgery is done to relieve stenosis, *both* kidneys are bombarded by the same pressure, so the "protected" one may deteriorate in the long run, unless the surgery worked well or unless drugs are used to lower the pressure. If *drugs* are used instead of surgery, the stenotic kidney may deteriorate, or even infarct, because it fails to receive enough blood. This is a real dilemma! Current evidence suggests that surgical treatment is more successful at preserving renal function than drug treatment.

PTA

The newest approach to treatment of renal artery stenosis is balloon dilatation, better called percutaneous transluminal angioplasty (PTA). In this procedure, a double-lumen catheter with a balloon near the tip is placed in the stenotic area by a radiologist, then inflated to squash the occluding plaque. Atherosclerotic lesions tend to recur after balloon dilatation, and thus we need to know more about long-term effects. However, PTA is a wonderful new alternative to surgery.

As it becomes more common, percutaneous transluminal angioplasty may replace surgery when the stenosis is readily accessible to catheters. It is definitely contraindicated when the artery is calcified or ulcerated or when the lesions are at artery branches. Complications of PTA have been surprisingly rare, only about 10% of the procedures are marred by things like clotting, bleeding, emboli, or renal deterioration. This incidence will undoubtedly diminish as operators gain skill and as less complex cases are dilated.

Summary

All known renal diseases account for only 5–10% of hypertension. Of these, about half are caused by abnormal vessels that surgery can repair (affecting the major arteries or affecting only one kidney).

It is possible that many more hypertensives have subtle abnormalities impairing renal sodium excretion; but if so, the abnormalities cannot be detected by current methods and could not be treated surgically.

Activation of the renin–angiotensin–aldosterone system and the kidneys' poor excretion of sodium *both* participate in raising pressure in most renal hypertension.

The simplest tests to screen for renovascular hypertension are auscultation, searching for a systolic–diastolic bruit, and a rapid-sequence IVP.

The best tests of the relative role of the renin system in renal hypertension are measurement of renal vein renin levels and testing the pressure change after administration of a blocker like captopril. These also offer prognostic indicators for the success of arterial repair by surgery or by percutaneous transluminal angioplasty.

5 Well-Understood Causes of Hypertension: II. Primary Hyperaldosteronism and Other Forms of Endocrine Hypertension

Introduction

Primary hyperaldosteronism is the obverse of renal artery stenosis: the renin–angiotensin–aldosterone system is stimulated, at the aldosterone end, by diseases residing in the adrenal gland itself. The term "primary" is used to differentiate these causes from the increased aldosterone secretion seen in renal artery stenosis, Bartter's Syndrome, and other conditions in which renin is elevated. The syndromes with abnormally *high renin* levels have "*secondary*" *hyperaldosteronism*—the increased aldosterone is "secondary" to increased renin secretion.

The known normal stimuli of aldosterone secretion are angiotensins II and III, ACTH, and high serum K^+ levels. (Recently, a protein factor originating in the pituitary gland has been found in human urine; this factor stimulates aldosterone secretion, but its nature is unknown.) In primary hyperaldosteronism, *none* of these stimuli is the cause, and none of them circulate in increased amounts.

Because cases of primary hyperaldosteronism involve an autonomous, hyperactive adrenal gland making lots of aldosterone and needing no encouragement from the renin–angiotensin system, THE PLASMA RENIN LEVELS ARE LOW. In adrenal diseases causing excess aldosterone secretion, renin secretion is suppressed by the effects of increased aldosterone (i.e., salt retention, fluid retention, and expansion of the blood volume).

Pathologic Classification of Adrenal Gland in Primary Hyperaldosteronism

Adrenal *adenoma* of the glomerulosa zone (Conn's Syndrome) usually occurs in one gland only. It is a tumor that is benign in behavior. This tumor causes two-thirds of the cases of primary hyperaldosteronism.

Adrenal *carcinoma* of the glomerulosa zone, malignant in behavior, is a rare tumor.

Adrenal *hyperplasia* involves the glomerulosa zones of both glands is the second most common cause of primary hyperaldosteronism.

1. Although this condition suggests that there is some stimulus driving the glomerulosa zone to hypertrophy and to hypersecrete, that stimulus is not known. Certainly, it is not renin–angiotensin, because their levels are low in this syndrome. It could reflect extraordinary sensitivity to classical stimuli (angiotensin, ACTH, or potassium) or to an as-yet-unknown stimuli.
2. Some people think that hyperplasia is the precursor of adenomas. In fact, in cases of hyperplasia, many little adenomas may dot the glands ("multinodular hyperplasia").
3. There is great disagreement over the frequency of this condition: Conn proposed that fully 25% of all hypertensives have adrenal glomerulosa hyperplasia; most people feel that it is closer to 2.5%.

Clinical Features of Primary Hyperaldosteronism

Laboratory Findings

Primary hyperaldosteronism is characterized by:

1. High aldosterone levels in blood (>10 ng/100 ml) and in urine (>20 μg/day). (These numbers vary from lab to lab, depending on methodology.)

2. Low plasma renin levels (despite upright posture, salt restriction, or diuretics, all of which should raise renin).
3. High urine potassium excretion. The kidney is stimulated by aldosterone to reabsorb sodium and excrete potassium in its place.
4. Low serum potassium. With time, the constant stimulus by aldosterone to reabsorb sodium and trade off potassium into the urine depletes the body of potassium. Most of the symptoms of primary hyperaldosteronism result from the effects of depleted potassium.
5. Note that since the effects of aldosterone are exerted on the distal tubule (a sort of "fine-tuning" of the sodium balance just before the urine is excreted) there would be *no* effects of aldosterone if *no sodium* ever reached the distal tubule! When patients are placed on very low salt diets, all of the sodium is reabsorbed in the proximal tubule and loop of Henle. There may then be no sodium reaching distal tubules, nothing for the aldosterone site to work on, and no loss of potassium. Thus, there *can be hyperaldosteronism without potassium depletion,* a confusing diagnostic picture!
6. Alkalosis. (Remember the term "Hypokalemic Alkalosis.") As potassium is lost in the urine under the influence of high aldosterone, some hydrogen ion goes with it, and more H^+ enters the cells to replace potassium. This leads to a lower H^+ concentration in the blood, or alkalosis.

History and Physical Exam

Patients with primary hyperaldosteronism display:

1. Hypertension. This is almost never malignant, but can be quite severe, with levels as high as 280/140 mm Hg.
2. Weakness. Apparently, the loss of potassium in the urine depletes potassium in the muscle as well as in the blood and causes muscle weakness.
3. Polyuria and nocturia. A low potassium level damages the renal tubules (Hypokalemic Nephropathy), impairing the ability to concentrate urine. As a result of this impairment, a profuse, dilute urine is excreted night and day.
4. There is *no edema* in primary hyperaldosteronism (unless heart failure or other diseases complicate the picture). Edema is a phenomenon of complex etiology. Despite the presence of fluid retention in hyperaldosteronism, there is no leakage of fluid into the tissue spaces. For one thing, long-term hyperaldosteronism can lead to "escape" of the kidneys from the fluid-retaining effects of aldosterone. Second, the total-body autoregulation that results from increased blood volume and

increased cardiac output may cause arteriolar vasoconstriction which in turn protects the capillaries from pressures that would otherwise cause them to leak.

Diagnostic Sequence

In screening large populations measure the following:

1. Serum potassium. Look for levels below 3.5 mEq/L. (About 20% of patients with primary aldosteronism will *not* have low serum potassium; they will pass through the screen.)
2. Urine potassium. Look for excretion over 60 mEq/day.

In pursuing suspicious cases measure the following:

1. Plasma aldosterone levels or 24-hr urinary excretion of aldosterone.
   a. Draw the plasma early in the morning. Normal people have higher aldosterone levels after 10 A.M., after they have been up and around and stimulated their renin secretion. This can lead to falsely positive diagnoses of hyperaldosteronism. By contrast, patients with adenomas seem to have lower aldosterone levels after they arise and walk around for a few hours than they have when they first awaken. So, if the sample is drawn too late, the patients with tumors may have lost their high levels, whereas the normals may have driven their low levels up.
   b. A slightly more complex diagnostic maneuver involves measuring plasma aldosterone before the patient arises in the morning and again after the patient has been up and walking for 2 hr. Normals exhibit a rise in aldosterone with upright posture, patients with adenomas exhibit a fall. Apparently, normal adrenal glomerulosa is responsive primarily to angiotensin, which is elevated by 2 hr of upright posture. By contrast, adenomas are more responsive to ACTH than to angiotensin, and ACTH falls during the passage of 2 hr of morning time.
   c. A more refined test involves drawing plasma aldosterone before and after an intravenous saline load, usually 2 L of normal saline infused in 4 hr. Normals turn off their aldosterone, tumors do not.
2. Plasma renin levels.
   a. Draw this after patients have been standing for 1 hr or longer. This would drive the renin up in normals; but when primary aldosteronism is present, renin stays low all day. A more refined test involves drawing plasma renin after diuretic administration. This

is hard to interpret unless the diuretic dose and the normal response have been standardized at your hospital.

3. ^{131}I-Labeled cholesterol scan.
   a. This test uses a radioactive derivative of cholesterol that localizes in the adrenal gland. It partially masquerades as the precursor of steroid biosynthesis but cannot be metabolized all the way to steroid, so it sticks in the gland, glowing in the dark. Tumors and hyperplastic glands stand out by virtue of their increased mass and increased steroid metabolism.
   b. Optimum interpretation of this test requires that patients have their adrenal fasciculata and reticuleris zones quieted with an ACTH-suppressing dose of exogenous steroid (e.g., dexamethasone, 2.0 mg) for 2 days before the scan. When this is done, only the relatively autonomous lesions continue to take up labeled cholesterol.
   c. This test best identifies solitary tumors.
4. Adrenal vein catheterization.
   a. A catheter threaded into the adrenal vein can sample venous blood in order to measure aldosterone levels. This is only valuable if both veins are sampled. Although analogous to renal vein catheterizations for renin levels, the entire procedure is harder, as the adrenal vein is smaller.
   b. Once a catheter is placed in the adrenal vein, radiographic dye can be forced retrograde into the gland. This depicts the veins and can display the outlines of a hyperplastic gland or a tumor. The maneuver can also cause hemorrhage in the gland and can result in adrenal infarcts. This test is used infrequently today.
5. Other tests.
   a. The CT scan can pick up some (but not all) tumors. Better machines will lead to greater accuracy in the future.
   b. Administration of spironolactone, a competitive antagonist of aldosterone, has been advocated as a "therapeutic trial" to reveal cases of hyperaldosteronism. Unfortunately, spironolactone at the recommended doses (200–400 mg/day) lowers the pressure in many hypertensives, with and without adrenal tumors. Thus, this test could only be recommended as a screening test of low discrimination, to be used in cases where laboratory measurements are hard to obtain.
6. Abbreviated diagnostic scheme for primary hyperaldosteronism:
   a. Serum K^+. Is it low? If so, collect urine.
   b. Urine K^+. Is it high? If so, draw plasma.

TABLE I

Practice Grid[a]

Clinical condition	*Blood volume*	*Aldo (in blood or urine)*	*Renin (in peripheral blood)*	*K^+ (blood)*	*K^+ (urine)*	*Na^+ (urine)*
Primary hyperaldosteronism						
Dehydration						
Licorice fetish[b]						
Cirrhosis with ascites						
Renal tubular defect causing Na^+ retention[c]						

[a] Answers are at the end of the book (p. 200).
[b] Licorice contains a salt-retaining substance, glycyrrhizinic acid.
[c] Liddle's Syndrome.

c. Plasma renin and aldosterone. If renin is low and aldosterone is high, try to localize the lesion with radiographic techniques, including the ^{131}I-labeled cholesterol scan and CT scan.
d. Scans. If no tumors show up, conclude that hyperplasia is present and treat with drugs, including K^+-sparing diuretics.

Many conditions have one or more of the features of primary aldosteronism. For example, other steroids with some mineralocorticoid activity (such as hydrocortisone) can cause hypertension and suppressed renin. However, the aldosterone levels in such cases would be low. The key to accurate diagnosis of primary aldosteronism is the presence of high aldosterone and low renin in the blood. As practice for answering questions about this syndrome, fill out the preceding grid (Table I). (More about low-renin essential hypertension in a subsequent section.)

Treatment

Surgery is the best treatment for solitary tumors, resulting in a cure of the hypertension in 70% of cases. The surgical cure rate in bilateral hyperplasia is only 20% (when subtotal adrenalectomy is performed).

Medical treatment of inoperable tumor cases (and all cases of hyperplasia) involves the use of diuretics to reverse the sodium retention of excessive aldosterone, and of any other drugs that may be needed to control blood pressure.

The most specific diuretic for hyperaldosteronism is spironolactone (Aldactone), a competitive inhibitor of aldosterone. Its ratio of potency is about 1000 : 1, requiring 1 mg of drug to antagonize 1 μg of hormone. Thus, it may require doses of 400 mg/day to treat hyperaldosteronism. At those levels, spironolactone causes unpleasant side effects, such as nausea and gynecomastia in males and menstrual changes in females. If these symptoms occur, less spironolactone can be used together with other diuretics. Another alternative is the use of other "potassium-sparing" diuretics in place of spironolactone. In any event, the two goals of drug therapy are lowering of pressure and cessation of potassium loss.

Other Endocrine Causes of Hypertension

Congenital Adrenal Hyperplasia

These constitute a group of diseases, all hereditary and all marked by one of two different blocks in the enzymatic sequences normally leading to synthesis of hydrocortisone. In one form, 11-hydroxylation does not occur, and in another, 17-hydroxylation does not occur. Hydrocortisone synthesis requires both steps. The low levels of hydrocortisone caused by these inborn errors release the pituitary gland from suppression, and the ACTH level in the blood rises. ACTH stimulates the crippled adrenal cortex, which produces a great quantity of hydrocortisone precursors, some of which are salt retaining and some of which are androgenic. Depending on the specific enzyme defect, patients with congenital adrenal hyperplasia may have hypertension, masculinization, or lack of sexual development. These cases of hypertension usually arise in childhood and resemble primary hyperaldosteronism in many respects, including low serum potassium levels.

Unlike the situation in primary hyperaldosteronism, hypertension accompanying congenital adrenal hyperplasia responds to treatment with a glucocorticoid. The exogenous steroid turns off ACTH production, the abnormal steroid excesses subside, excessive salt is diuresed, and pressure falls to normal. A trial of oral dexamethasone, testing its effect on blood pressure, can be a useful diagnostic maneuver. Better yet, measure plasma and urine *aldosterone levels*. These are *low* in congenital adrenal hyperplasia.

Cushing's Syndrome

Cushing's Syndrome can be caused by a variety of conditions, but it is always marked by excessive blood levels of *gluco*corticoids, such as hydrocortisone. The syndrome includes a long list of signs and symptoms, such as "moon-face," "purple striae" on the abdomen, high blood sugar, and high blood pressure. There are two components to the hypertension associated with Cushing's Syndrome: (1) excessive *mineralo*corticoid activity (because endogenous adrenal steroids have some mineralocorticoid activity) and (2) a second component caused by glucocorticoids. The second component of hypertension in Cushing's Syndrome includes *vasoconstriction* and *high cardiac output*. Vasoconstriction may result from *potentiation of catecholamine action* by glucocorticoids. Cardiac output may be increased by the action of glucocorticoids directly on the heart. This condition can be diagnosed by measuring plasma and urine glucocorticoid levels, which are high.

Other Endocrine Forms of Hypertension

Hyperthyroidism

This is the classical example of "high-output hypertension." Cardiac output is dramatically increased, largely because the pulse rate is increased. Peripheral resistance is decreased in most cases of hyperthyroidism. The skin feels warm. As a result of increased cardiac output and decreased peripheral resistance, the systolic pressure is increased, while the diastolic is decreased. (However, some patients also display a moderate increase in diastolic pressure.)

Thyroxine increases the number of β-adrenergic receptors. This potentiates the effects of circulating catecholamines. Most of the visible signs of hyperthyroidism are the result of this action, and can be blocked by β-adrenergic blockers (such as propranolol). Certainly, the hypertension associated with hyperthyroidism is a result of excessive catecholamine activity; it disappears with administration of β blockers. Of course, treatment of the increased thyroid activity also alleviates the hypertension.

Hypothyroidism

For reasons that remain obscure, about 25% of patients with hypothyroidism have diastolic hypertension. (Part of this group may simply have essential hypertension.) Of these patients, about one-third will revert to normal blood pressure when their hypothyroidism is treated with thyroxine.

Unlike patients with hyperthyroidism, those with myxedema (hypothyroidism) have increased peripheral resistance and tend to be volume depleted. They look like patients trying to retain their body heat and fluids. On treatment with thyroid hormone, their vessels and kidneys open up.

Hyperparathyroidism

For reasons that are absolutely unfathomable, people with hyperparathyroidism have an increased incidence of hypertension. There is growing interest in the role of calcium in blood pressure regulation, but no clear picture has emerged.

Acromegaly

About one in three acromegalics have hypertension. There is apparent sodium retention in acromegaly. Treatment of the underlying disease results in normalization of blood pressure. It could be that growth hormone is one of the mysterious pituitary factors that stimulate aldosterone secretion.

Summary

The constellation of high pressure and high aldosterone, low renin, and low potassium levels in the blood is pathognomonic of primary hyperaldosteronism. Other endocrine syndromes with hypertension may have one or two of these abnormal laboratory findings, but not all three.

6 Well-Understood Causes of Hypertension: III. Pheochromocytomas

Introduction

Pheochromocytomas (commonly called ''pheo's'') are rare tumors that secrete either *epinephrine* or *norepinephrine,* the two major *catecholamines* made in the body that can elevate blood pressure. (Dopamine is the third major catecholamine, but its effects on blood pressure are minimal.) Pheochromocytomas are the cause of hypertension in no more than 1 out of 1000 patients with high blood pressure.

People with pheochromocytomas exhibit signs and symptoms that are exaggerations of the normal ''fight-or-flight'' reaction, including rapid pulse, elevated blood pressure, apprehension, sweating, and elevated blood glucose. Although these features would help save an animal or human confronted with mortal danger, they can cause more harm than good when repeated or sustained.

The original classification of the *adrenergic* (*sympathetic*) *nervous system* divided the sympathetic nervous system into those parts producing *epi-*

nephrine (adrenaline) and those parts producing *norepinephrine* (noradrenaline). The adrenal medulla is the only organ that can make epinephrine. The medulla can also make norepinephrine; the sympathetic nerves make only norepinephrine.

The more modern classification divides the sympathetic system on the basis of its receptors, α and β (plus the dopaminergic receptors in kidney and brain).

1. α-Adrenergic receptors mediate constriction of vessels and dilation of pupils. The classical transmitter is norepinephrine.
2. β-Adrenergic receptors mediate selective dilation of vessels (in muscle), dilation of the bronchioles, increased cardiac contraction and rate, and formation of glucose from glycogen. The endogenous β transmitter is epinephrine, although norepinephrine exerts β effects in addition to its well-known α effects.

The metabolism of catecholamines can be described in the following manner:

1. Norepinephrine gives rise to epinephrine in the adrenal medulla.
2. *Met*hylation in the liver or kidney creates nor*met*anephrine and *met*anephrine (from norepinephrine and epinephrine, respectively).
3. The *metanephrines* can be conjugated and excreted in the urine or further metabolized.
4. Removal of the amino group leads to synthesis of *vanillylmandelic acid* (VMA). (Since the amino group is the site of attachment of the methyl group that distinguishes epinephrine from norepinephrine, the absence of the amino group removes that distinction, and VMA is the *common metabolic product* of both catecholamines.)

Pathology

Pheochromocytomas are tumors derived from chromaffin cells of the sympathetic nervous systems and from some other cells of neural crest origin.

Most pheochromocytomas develop in the adrenal medulla (two-thirds), some are found elsewhere in the abdominal sympathetic chains (one-third), and a very few arise in the bladder, neck, chest, ear, eye, etc.

Most pheochromocytomas are single and benign, but a few are malignant and metastatic.

There are some pheochromocytomas that are *benign,* but *multiple!* The multiple, benign ones are often part of a *familial* syndrome called Multiple Endocrine Adenomatosis, Type II, or Sipple's Syndrome. This includes pheochromocytomas, medullary carcinoma of the thyroid producing calcitonin, and occasional tumors of the parathyroid glands.

Some families have an inherited tendency to pheochromocytomas *without* other endocrine tumors.

About 10% of patients with Von Recklinghausen's Disease (neurofibromatosis) have pheochromocytomas.

Pathophysiology of Hypertension in Pheochromocytoma

Pheochromocytomas originating in the adrenal medulla make epinephrine; those originating elsewhere make norephinephrine. This heterogeneous origin leads to a heterogeneity of clinical pictures. Pheochromocytomas producing epinephrine cause more apprehension and tachycardia for a given amount of hypertension, whereas those producing norepinephrine cause more hypertension and relatively less of the associated symptoms.

The elevated blood pressure in pheochromocytoma almost certainly results from a combination of increases in the two classic components of pressure: *cardiac output* and *peripheral resistance*. Catecholamines also affect the kidneys, reducing their ability to excrete salt and water, so the Guyton mechanism may be active in this disease.

Clinical Features

History and Physical Examination

The history and physical examination may reveal the following clinical features in a patient with a pheochromocytoma.

1. *Hypertension:* primarily systolic in epinephrine secretors, and systolic plus diastolic in norepinephrine secretors.
2. *Paroxysms* of
   a. Hypertension
   b. Headache
   c. Sweating
   d. Palpitations
   e. Nervousness
   f. Nausea and vomiting

   Paroxysms of catecholamine release and hypertension can be provoked by a variety of stimuli, such as smoking, drugs, exercise, fear, pregnancy, (and fear of pregnancy!).

The problem with the symptomatic diagnosis of pheochromocytoma is the almost universal occurrence of episodes of headaches, nervousness, sweating and/or palpitations. It is easy to evoke from any hypertensive a history of episodic symptoms. Yet pheochromocytomas are extremely rare. The diagnosis really depends on laboratory confirmation.

3. Paradoxical *falls* in blood pressure are also seen in patients with pheo.
   a. First, these patients have extreme lability of many parameters—sometimes up, sometimes down.
   b. Second, the periods of high pressure can result in the excretion of increased sodium and fluid by the kidney, causing *reduced blood volume*. With a small blood volume, these patients are susceptible to drops in blood pressure between spurts of catecholamine secretion.
   c. Finally, the catecholamines stimulate both α- and β-adrenergic receptors. The β-receptors cause dilation of some blood vessels (the ones a frightened animal would need to escape, especially the vessels of the muscles). Thus, release of mostly epinephrine, in contrast to norepinephrine, would cause some vasodilation, contributing to a drop in pressure.

Laboratory Tests

The best test for pheochromocytoma is measurement of *plasma catecholamines*.

1. The sample must be drawn when the patient is lying down and resting, for example, first thing in the morning before the patient arises from bed.
2. Anything as traumatic as a needle-stick will cause a burst of catecholamines to be released into the blood; therefore, the blood for this test must be drawn through an indwelling needle or catheter (e.g., a "heparin well") that has been inserted 30 min or more before the test.
3. Normal values are about 0.5 ng/ml. Patients with tumors have values above 1.0 ng/ml.
4. This test usually measures total catecholamine levels. In some laboratories the individual catecholamines can be characterized. (Such a fractionation could help to localize the tumor, since epinephrine-secreting tumors are almost always in the abdomen.)

The second-best test for pheochromocytoma is measurement of *urinary metanephrines*.

1. This test measures the first metabolites of catecholamines formed outside the tumor.

2. To correct for time and for the completeness of urine collection, the excretion is expressed "per milligram creatinine." Creatinine is excreted at a fairly constant rate all day. The average adult excretes 1 gm/day. When only one voiding, or less than a day's output of urine is collected, measuring the creatinine in that sample will tell what proportion of a day's output is in the collection.
3. Normals excrete about 1 μg metanephrines per mg creatinine (or 1 mg/day). Patients with pheochromocytomas excrete more than 2 μg/mg of creatinine (or 2 mg/day).
4. There is recent evidence that the *metanephrines excreted during sleep* are better discriminators between tumors and normals than a 24-hr collection.

A quick-and-dirty test for pheochromocytoma is measurement of *urinary VMA* (vanillylmandelic acid), the end product of catecholamine metabolism. This is a measure of the sum of all catecholamines.

1. This test is imprecise and should be discontinued. Many normals have high values, and many patients with tumor have low values.
2. The normal value is less than 6.5 mg/day.

Drugs and foods can interfere with the tests for pheochromocytoma.

1. Obviously, vanilla interferes with the accurate measurement of catecholamines based on vanillylmandelic acid. So do bananas, coffee, or chocolate.
2. Even more obviously, the ingestion or inhalation of drugs containing catecholamines will foul up a catecholamine assays (e.g., aerosols for asthma and nasal decongestants).
3. As will be described later, many drugs used in therapy of hypertension affect the autonomic nervous system and can affect excretion of catecholamines. Chief offenders are methyldopa (Aldomet®) and reserpine.
4. Not-so-obvious are problems encountered in the laboratory because of interference by phenothiazines, tetracyclines, and alcohol.

Blood Sugar Measurements

Because of the effect of catecholamines on liver and muscle glycogen, blood glucose is elevated during paroxysms of symptoms and hypertension in patients with pheochromocytoma. However, because it is so difficult to catch a patient during a paroxysm, the measurement of blood sugar is only useful in about half of the cases.

"Provocative" Tests

Since most pheochromocytomas secrete only sporadically, diagnosis may depend on the use of provocative tests, in which a substance is injected that would stimulate secretion by a tumor, but not by a normal adrenal gland.

Today, the best provocateur is the hormone glucagon. Apparently, pheochromocytomas have receptors for glucagon, a hormone that stimulates the release of catecholamines.

To do the test:

1. Start iv or insert indwelling catheter into vein. Wait 30 min.
2. Make sure you have phentolamine (Regitine) handy for iv use to block the released catecholamines if they should cause a dangerous rise in pressure. (More about phentolamine later.)
3. Draw control blood and mark the tube **control!**
4. Give 2 mg of glucagon iv by bolus (push) infusion.
5. Draw blood for plasma catecholamines about 2 min after injecting glucagon. Mark the tube!
6. Measure blood pressure every 60 sec for about 5 min before and after the test.
7. The test is positive if blood pressure rises by 30/15 mm Hg (30 mm systolic, 15 mm diastolic). Usually, positive tests are even more striking.
8. The test is positive if plasma catecholamine levels rise into a clearly abnormal range (2 ng/ml), or triple their control levels.

This test can be dangerous! A sudden burst of high pressure is more damaging to the body than chronic elevation. Use this test only if your index of suspicion is high, if plasma catecholamines or urinary metanephrines are not available, if resting pressure is near normal, and if iv phentolamine is at-the-ready.

Confusing Features

The paroxysmal nature of the symptoms and hypertension in some cases of pheochromocytoma makes it easy to miss the diagnosis. Many normals have wide fluctuations, and experience with these lulls the observer into ignoring sporadic symptoms in a *bona fide* pheo patient.

Problems with cross-reacting chemicals can easily foul up the laboratory diagnosis.

There is poor correlation between lab values and the level of blood pressure. Even in proven cases, the pressure can either be surprisingly high or surprisingly low compared to the catecholamine values. This discrepancy may be caused by variable blood-volume depletion (mentioned earlier), the presence of β-adrenergic influence with its attendant vasodilatation, or the release of prostaglandins or other vasodilators in response to bursts of catecholamines.

Tumor Localization

Pheochromocytomas are most commonly found by accident in a routine *intravenous pyelogram* (IVP). Suspicious findings can be supplemented by tomograms (radiographic slices). The clue is displacement of a kidney or defects in its silhouette.

There is a growing use of the *CT scanner* to find pheochromocytomas. This will be the best localizing test in the future.

Arteriography, deliberately designed to find a pheochromocytoma or performed to look for renal artery stenosis, can localize pheochromocytomas.

Drawing venous blood samples through a catheter in the *inferior vena cava* can help localization. The catheter is advanced from the lumbar region to the right atrium, with blood being drawn at about six levels. This can help find tumors that cannot be seen, especially recurrent tumors after prior excisions.

Radioactive catecholamine analogs are being developed for localization of pheochromocytomas by *nuclear medicine* techniques. They may be extremely useful for either small tumors or for those in unusual locations. It is easy to scan a whole human looking for "hot spots" where an isotope has localized.

Therapy

An untreated pheochromocytoma is usually fatal. Complete surgical removal of the tumor is the definitive treatment. The problems encountered in the surgical approach include (1) the prevention of dramatic hypertension during the surgery itself and (2) the unexpected existence of more than one tumor. Second or third tumors can be as far removed from the usual location in the abdomen as the neck!

Drugs can prepare the patient for surgery, and they can be used in inoperable cases. Best suited for this preparation are α-adrenergic blockers, such as phentolamine (Regitine®) or phenoxybenzamine (Dibenzyline®). Prazosin (Minipress®) is a newer blocker that is easy to use.

β-Blockers such as propranolol (Inderal®) can be useful if added to α blockers, but the use of β blockers alone is risky: they might block the vasodilatation caused by β receptors and expose pure vasocontriction caused by the α receptors. *Never give β blockers before α blockers* in pheochromocytoma! In fact, if *any* patient with hypertension exhibits an unexpected rise in pressure when given a β blocker (or guanethidine), it is a good idea to look for a pheochromocytoma. This paradoxical response can be a helpful clue to the presence of pheos.

Summary

Pheochromocytomas are very rare tumors that cause episodic adrenergic symptoms superimposed on a picture of fairly constant hypertension.

The best diagnostic tests for pheochromocytoma are the measurement of plasma catecholamines in resting patients and the localization of tumors by CT scan.

Although rare (1 in 1000 hypertensives), pheochromocytomas are frequently fatal if undiscovered and capable of establishing a new physician's reputation if successfully removed.

7 Well-Understood Causes of Hypertension: IV. Coarctation of the Aorta

Anatomy

Coarctation is a narrowing that impedes the flow of blood through the aorta. It causes elevated pressure proximal to the lesion, but not distal to it. The constriction can occur anywhere along the aorta. More proximal lesions cause problems earlier and are usually evident in infancy. Cases that turn up after 1 year of age are usually characterized by constriction further down the aorta. Severe cases are usually accompanied by other congenital cardiac defects. For example, girls with Turner's Syndrome have a high incidence of coarctation.

Pathophysiology of Hypertension in Coarctation

There is obviously increased resistance to arterial flow caused by the narrowed aorta. In addition, there is a contribution from the renin–angiotensin system, which is activated by relative ischemia in the kidneys below the constriction. In a way, coarctation is analogous to bilateral renal artery stenosis.

Diagnosis

Diagnosis is facilitated by the fact that arterial *pressure is higher in the arms than the legs* or in one arm compared to the other. (Normally, thigh pressure is slightly higher than pressure in the arms.) Also, the pulse pressure is narrowed in the legs. Some astute clinicians can feel a delay in the pulse between the wrist and ankle.

Every person who measures blood pressure should have a large cuff for his/her sphygmomanometer and should *measure the pressure in the legs of every hypertensive child and young adult at least once!* The cuff is applied around the thigh and the sounds of Korotkoff can be heard behind the knee.

The murmur caused by the coarctation itself can be heard over the chest, both front and back, during systole.

A history of pain or weakness in the legs during exercise is sometimes given.

The chest X ray is often diagnostic with two features:

1. "3" sign (a dent along the right-hand edge of the profile of the aorta)
2. Notching of the ribs (caused by enlarged intercostal vessels that act as collaterals around the coarct)

Prognosis

After 1 year of age, survivors have a 1-in-4 chance of dying in the next 20 years, then a 1-in-2 chance during each successive 20 years. In other words, there is an early mortality peak in the first year, a relative grace period during childhood, and a bad prognosis for the adult years.

The usual causes of death from coarcts are heart failure, ruptured aorta, bacterial endocarditis, and stroke.

The hypertension of coarctation is *not* likely to become "malignant" (see Chapter 22), probably because the kidneys in this disease are always "protected" from the beating they usually take from high blood pressure. This is analogous to the "protected" kidney behind a renal artery stenosis.

Treatment

There is only one definitive treatment—vascular surgery. Surgery is much more successful if done early in life. Frequently, there is a long gap in the medical surveillance of individuals between the pediatric age group and those entering the ranks of the army, college, or the insured! This can stand in the way of early disease detection. We must find coarcts *early*. After surgery, about 30% of people who have had coarctation remain hypertensive. This is partly the result of already damaged vessels, and partly the result of the natural incidence of hypertension.

8 Well-Understood Causes of Hypertension: V. Estrogens and Other Drugs

Introduction

The widespread use of estrogens both in birth control pills and to relieve symptoms of menopause makes "The Pill" *the most common reversible cause of hypertension*. Certainly, simply stopping The Pill in women with estrogen-induced hypertension is the easiest of all the treatments for high blood pressure.

Although all women taking estrogens for birth control or menopause are likely to have a rise in systolic and diastolic blood pressure, it usually amounts to only 5–10 mm Hg, and only a minority of women develop significant hypertension. Whether the effect of estrogens on pressure is slight or great it takes about 9 months to reach a maximum.

Incidence of Significant Hypertension with Estrogens

Only about 5% of all women on estrogens will become frankly hypertensive in the first year, and some become severely hypertensive. Why this small fraction of patients experiences more than the customary 5–10 mm rise in pressure is unknown.

The incidence of hypertension among women on estrogens increases with time. After 5 years, as many as 15% are hypertensive. This is more than the expected increase in hypertension seen in all adults with aging.

Estrogen-related hypertension is more common in women over 35, and *much more* common in those over 45. Obesity or a family history of hypertension increases the odds of becoming hypertensive with estrogens. The hypertension associated with oral contraceptive estrogens probably contributes to their known tendency to aggravate cardiovascular disease and stroke.

Pathophysiology of Hypertension with Estrogens

The mechanism of estrogen-induced hypertension is probably a combination of three factors:

1. The sodium-retaining properties of estrogenic steroids, causing increased blood volume and increased cardiac output.
2. Elevation of renin substrate concentration, with consequent increase in renin activity and angiotensin production. Angiotensin increases aldosterone production and vasoconstriction. This rise in renin *activity* occurs despite a reflex fall in renin *enzyme* release [i.e., plasma renin *activity* (PRA) is up despite the fact that plasma renin *concentration* (PRC) is down].
3. Estrogens potentiate the actions of catecholamines, largely by inducing an increased number of catecholamine receptors.

Management

Carry out regular blood pressure checks before and after starting estrogens for either contraception or treatment of the menopause; these should be mandatory. Check the pressure every 3–6 months for 1 year and then annually.

Withdraw estrogens from those suffering significant rises in pressure. (We will discuss later the degree of elevation that constitutes "significance.") Do not make a final judgment about the role played by estrogens until at least *6 months* after stopping them. Elevated pressure can take that long to come back down. If the pressure stays up despite discontinuing estrogens, it is theoretically reasonable to start them again if the need persists (e.g., menopause, severe osteoporosis, or contraception). If that is done, the hypertension must be treated with standard therapy.

Treat the residual hypertension in those whose pressure fails to return to normal after stopping estrogens. Up to half of the patients will not revert to normal pressure after the steroid is stopped. (This is simply a restatement of the recommendation to treat all hypertension.)

Offer an alternative means of birth control. Pregnancy is a cardiovascular risk in its own right (not to mention the possible ramifications of unwanted pregnancy).

Suggest the use of birth control pills containing only progestational steroids (the "mini pill"); they may not be as hypertensive, depending on the progestin used. Pure progesterone is a diuretic and should *lower* pressure, but some synthetic progestins have mineralocorticoid (aldosterone-like) actions.

Other Drugs That Cause Hypertension

Alcohol

The intake of more than three drinks per day is associated with increased blood pressure. The higher the intake, the higher the pressure. The mechanism of this rise in unknown, but cessation of alcohol leads to a fall of pressure back to normal.

During the withdrawal or "detoxification" stage *after* chronic alcohol ingestion, there is a burst of elevated pressure that can be alarming. It looks very much like an attack of pheochromocytoma or a giant catecholamine release. In general, sedation is the only treatment needed (e.g., chlordiazepoxide, Librium®); the hypertensive attack will pass, along with the other manifestations or withdrawal. There has been a flurry of interest in the drug clonidine (Catepres®) for treatment of withdrawals from a variety of addicting drugs. It reduces catecholamine output by its central nervous system effects. This may be a useful drug for alcohol withdrawal hypertension.

Amphetamines and Nasal Decongestants

Drugs that mimic or stimulate the adrenergic nervous system can raise blood pressure to alarming heights. They were popular during the wars for men who wanted to avoid the draft by feigning hypertension. They can be particularly dangerous in *bona fide* hypertensives who are intrinsically hypersensitive to catecholamines. Such patients should be warned about that danger. The major problem is knowing which of the easily available cold remedies have sympathomimetic drugs in them. Since most do, to treat allergic or cold symptoms in hypertensives, one should prescribe drugs such as aspirin or antihistaminics, in formulations that do not contain sympathomimetic drugs.

9 Well-Understood Causes of Hypertension: VI. Pregnancy and Preeclampsia-Eclampsia

Normal Pregnancy and Blood Pressure

The average woman who becomes pregnant has a slight fall in arterial blood pressure (5–10 mm) by the eighth month. This returns to control levels by the time of delivery.

Pressure during pregnancy is lowest when women lie on their left side. Rolling over onto the back results in a rise of 10–15 mm, probably caused by the weight of the uterus on the kidneys or vessels, followed by release of a pressor hormone or a reflex sympathetic discharge.

In normal pregnancy, renin substrate, renin activity (PRA), and aldosterone levels all rise markedly (about eightfold).

Normally, vessels become unresponsive to angiotensin during pregnancy, so blood pressure does not rise despite the rise in angiotensin (renin) levels. This may be the result of prostaglandins produced by the uteroplacental unit. (Apparently the adrenal glomerulosa continues to respond appropriately to angiotensin and produces large quantities of aldosterone.)

In normal pregnancy, the kidneys do not retain as much sodium as one would predict from the high aldosterone levels. Probably, a combination of prostaglandins and progesterone exert diuretic effects that antagonize aldosterone in the kidneys.

Preeclampsia and Eclampsia (Also Called "Toxemia")

Characterization

Preeclampsia is characterized by one or more of the following:

1. Hypertension
2. Edema
3. Proteinuria

Any one of these abnormalities is associated with increased risk of fetal damage, maternal morbidity, and the subsequent development of eclampsia itself.

Eclampsia is a combination of hypertension, proteinuria, edema **and** the following:

1. Convulsions, and
2. Coma, or
3. Death

Etiology

The only thing known for sure about the cause of eclampsia is that it arises in the uteroplacental unit. Delivery is followed promptly by reversal of the disease.

A commonly mentioned feature, *under-perfusion* of the uteroplacental unit, may come before or after the disease. If it comes before, the analogy to hypertension accompanying renal under-perfusion is tempting. However, there is no firm evidence for a circulating pressor released by the uterus or placenta.

Epidemiology

The disease is more common in women who

1. Are relatively young or old to be pregnant
2. Are having their first baby
3. Are having twins
4. Are having an abnormal pregnancy (such as hydatidiform mole)
5. Are obese

6. Have diabetes
7. Have a genitourinary infection
8. Are the daughters of women who had preeclampsia themselves

Pathogenesis

In contrast to women with a normal pregnancy, those with preeclampsia are unusually sensitive to angiotensin or norepinephrine.

There is marked increase in peripheral resistance. (Many vessels show pathological changes similar to those seen in malignant hypertension. These will be described in Chapter 11.)

Renal blood flow and glomerular filtration are decreased. The renal glomerular vessels show characteristic thickening and subendothelial deposits.

The increased pressure observed in preeclampsia could result from any one of the above changes, but probably results from a combination of them all. (The heart is clearly *not* involved in causing the high pressure. If anything, cardiac output goes *down*.)

The complications of eclampsia include fetal prematurity and deformity and both infant and maternal death. In fact, among all *definable* causes of fetal death, preeclampsia and eclampsia account for one in four (twice as common as *abruptio placenta* and five times as common as birth trauma). It is also the leading cause of prematurity (one in three premature deliveries is marked by preeclampsia).

Diagnosis

The most common diagnostic confusion is between preeclampsia and hypertension during pregnancy in a woman who has had hypertension *before* she became pregnant. This can sometimes be clarified by looking for signs of long-standing hypertension, such as an enlarged heart. Such signs favor the diagnosis of preexisting hypertension aggravated by pregnancy.

Furthermore, pregnancy-aggravated hypertension usually occurs *early* in gestation, whereas eclampsia arises after the fifth month.

Finally, it is perfectly possible to have true preeclampsia in a woman who *had* hypertension when she became pregnant.

The "roll-over test" may be helpful. Women destined to become preeclamptic have an exaggerated pressor response to rolling onto their backs from the left lateral recumbent position. (This test may be the equivalent of an endogenous angiotensin infusion secondary to pressure on the kidneys.) A positive test result is a rise of 20 mm or more in diastolic pressure within 10 min, especially in women beyond the 28th week of pregnancy.

Treatment

Bed rest, favoring the left lateral recumbent posture, is the cornerstone of treatment. It is both safe and inexpensive.

Reserve antihypertensive drugs for those women with extreme elevations in pressure. If drugs are needed, use vasodilators. Some other drugs, such as diuretics that lower plasma volume, can reduce perfusion of the uteroplacental unit even further than the disease does and may cause increased incidence of fetal damage. In one study, patients receiving diuretics had less successful pregnancies in terms of fetal health than those treated without diuretics. This study has been disputed, but it may be prudent to avoid diuretics if possible in pregnancy. We will discuss treatment again in a later chapter.

Treat convulsions with magnesium sulfate injections, and immediate delivery of the infant. This is a true medical emergency. (See chapter on Hypertensive Emergencies.)

Summary of Curable Causes of Hypertension

This list can be recalled by using the mnemonic RECAP:

1. *R*ENAL diseases, including renal artery stenosis
2. *E*STROGENS, including medications and pregnancy
3. *C*OARCTATION of the aorta
4. *A*LDOSTERONISM
5. *P*HEOCHROMOCYTOMA

Five other identifiable causes can be remembered by the letters A to E:

1. *A*LCOHOL excess or withdrawal
2. *B*RAIN lesions, including increased intracranial pressure
3. *C*USHING'S syndrome
4. *D*RUGS with sympathomimetic qualities
5. *E*XCESSIVE secretion of THYROID OR PARATHYROID hormone

10 Essential Hypertension

Introduction

This chapter describes the hypertension we see most often (95% of all cases) but fails to describe its cause—which is unknown. Most of the description is epidemiologic and statistical. Despite our prodigious research efforts and reasonably successful therapy, we still do not understand this disease very well.

Definitions (What is it?)

"Essential Hypertension" is simply hypertension of unknown cause. It is also called "Primary Hypertension." "Secondary Hypertension" is the elevated pressure that accompanies known causes, such as primary hyperaldosteronism, renal disease, and coarctation. Of all hypertension, 95% is essential, only 5% is secondary to known causes.

The difference between normal and hypertensive blood pressure is arbitrarily defined.

1. Life expectancy is inversely proportional to arterial pressure, either systolic, diastolic, or mean. (This relationship refers only to pressures above "shock" levels. Obviously, extremely low pressures are incompatible with life.)
2. There is no clear "break" in the curve that describes the relationship between pressure and mortality. There is no level below which pressure makes *no* difference, so *all* pressure is somewhat damaging.
3. Although a statistical definition could be derived from the pressures of the population as a whole, hypertension is most practically defined at levels where treatment will do more good than harm. (If a simple, safe pill or public water additive could lower blood pressure without side effects, *everyone* would probably benefit from it and 120/80 mm Hg, the current norm, could be considered too high.)

The average pressure of a population tends to rise with age (in developed countries). Therefore hypertension has been defined at higher pressure levels in older people. However, a closer look shows that some people *never* experience a rise in pressure with age, so the mean for a population is composed of a group of normotensives who do not change and a group of hypertensives who worsen with time. The old habit of discounting higher pressure in older people should be abandoned.

High pressure is more damaging to males than to premenopausal females; therefore, hypertension is defined at lower pressures in males than in premenopausal females. Again, the logic is to define hypertension at levels where treatment can exert a benefit that outweighs risks.

A summary of arbitrary cut-off pressures (those causing a death rate 150% of "normal") in mm Hg is

1. Men under 45 years: 130/90
2. Men over 45 years: 140/95
3. Women over 45 years: 140/95
4. Using these levels, about 10–15% of American adults have hypertension. Of these hypertensives, 70% have diastolic pressures under 105.
5. Remember, *either* systolic *or* diastolic pressure over these limits is "abnormal."
6. If you cannot tolerate a death rate 150% of "normal" in your patients or family (or self), then the pressures listed above are too high, and hypertension will be diagnosed at lower pressures.

Epidemiology (Who gets it?)

The *frequency* (or *incidence*) of hypertension is related to the following parameters:

1. *Age*. Above 60 years of age, 30% of white Americans and 50% of black Americans have pressures over 160/95.
2. *Sex*. Below age 45, more men than women have hypertension. After menopause, this relative female immunity disappears.
3. *Race*. At all ages and for both sexes, a higher percentage of American blacks have hypertension than American whites.
4. *Weight*. Obese people are more likely to be hypertensive. (In addition, the pressure is apt to be read incorrectly high when the cuff is too small for the fat arm. Even taking this artifact into account, obese people have more hypertension.)
5. *Salt intake*. The incidence of hypertension correlates with sodium intake when different nations or groups are compared. The relationship of pressure to salt intake in individuals is less dramatic. Recently, it has been found that blood pressure varies *inversely* with *potassium* intake. A high intake of potassium apparently lowers pressure! Most food processing not only adds sodium, it removes potassium, so many of the correlations with added sodium in the diet may have been inadvertent correlations with the absence of potassium! Potassium supplements cause mild diuresis in humans. Perhaps potassium's protective effect is exerted via the kidney.
6. *Heredity*. There is clearly a contribution to blood pressure from heredity. Even within families, people have a ''rank'' in their pressures, a rank that can be discerned in infancy and which persists throughout life (''tracking''). Roughly speaking, about 50% of the average hypertensive patient's *elevation* in pressure is determined genetically and 50% environmentally. This has been clearly demonstrated by studies of identical twins raised in different homes. (If we had to choose the one aspect of the *environment* that contributed most to hypertension, it would be dietary *salt*.)
    a. This implies that ''clean living'' and a healthy diet cannot *cure* high pressure, but only ameliorate it or delay its onset in patients with a genetic predisposition.
    b. By the same token, foul habits and high-salt diets will not do much to raise pressure in those who are constitutionally resistant to hypertension.
    c. Hypertension is apparently determined by many genes (polygenic), so it is difficult to predict with precision its occurrence in individual children of hypertensive adults.

7. *Other.* There is some evidence of correlations between hypertension and *extreme occupational stress, high alcohol intake* (more than three drinks per day), uterine *fibroids,* and *gout.* These are weak correlations. (Smoking and coffee apparently do not raise pressure except transiently. Even excessive use of cigarettes and coffee has no significant effect on basal blood pressure. Certainly, these habits do not, by themselves, cause fixed elevations of pressure.)

The *harmful effects* of hypertension are also regulated by some epidemiologic variables:

1. *Race.* At any given pressure, blacks suffer the ill effects of hypertension more than whites (especially stroke and renal failure). This affects the decision about when to treat.
2. *Genetics.* This helps determine the damage caused by high blood pressure in ways not yet understood. Whole families can carry extremely high pressures for normal life spans. (However, it may be that they would live still *longer* with *lower* pressures!)
3. *Other risk factors.* Although death and disease from atherosclerosis occur more frequently in hypertensives, the damage caused by hypertension is aggravated by other things that contribute to atherosclerosis. The other risk factors include *obesity, smoking, high blood lipids,* and *glucose intolerance* (see Fig. 3, p. 110). Each additional risk factor *multiples* the risk! Thus, people with moderate hypertension are *twice* as likely as normals to die of cardiovascular problems. If they also smoke, they are *four* times as likely to die, etc.

Classification of Essential Hypertension

Labile Hypertension

Labile hypertension is defined as the presence in one patient of normal and abnormal pressures at different examinations, with no evidence of target organ damage (i.e., no disease of heart, brain, eye, or kidney). Since *everyone* can experience an elevation of pressure given the appropriate stimulus, this entity has very diffuse borders. There is no clear demarcation between labile hypertension and normalcy.

Only about 5% of young, labile hypertensives progress to *sustained* hypertension (also called "fixed"). Labile hypertension is not particularly dangerous, and patients should not get excited about it. (That would only make them *more* labile!)

Labile hypertension occurs more frequently in males.

Labile hypertension is characterized by high cardiac output (rather than a high peripheral resistance).

Although bona fide hypertension can still be "labile" in its fluctuations around an elevated mean, this is NOT the common understanding of the term "labile hypertension." Most people think of it as *high* pressures occurring only *part* of the time, alternating with *normal* pressure.

Borderline Hypertension

This is the grey zone between clearly normal and clearly abnormal levels. The exact levels will vary, of course, as the definition of hypertension varies.

Sustained ("Fixed" or "Established") Hypertension

This is the most common type of hypertension, defined as exceeding the norm on three consecutive measurements (three different days).

Malignant Hypertension

This category of hypertension is also called "accelerated." (See Chapters 11 and 22.) This condition is marked by rapidly rising pressure, hemorrhages and exudates in the retina, protein in the urine, and—most dire—neurological changes that result from cerebral vasospasm, edema, and hemorrhage.

Evolution of Hypertension in Individuals

Early Picture

In its early stages, hypertension is characterized by relatively *high cardiac output* and normal peripheral resistance.

β-Adrenergic hyperactivity can be documented in many young hypertensives, but not in old ones.

Hypertension may not advance beyond this stage. In a small number of patients hypertension persists as a high-output form of hypertension. These patients form a subgroup of adult hypertensives called "*hyperkinetic*" or "*hyperdynamic*."

When large groups of patients were studied for long periods of times, many of those destined to develop sustained hypertension had higher pressures than their peers *as early as one month of age*, and they stayed ahead of their peers throughout life. (This process is called "tracking," and emphasizes the role of heredity in hypertension.)

Most people destined to have essential hypertension have clearly abnormal pressures in their *thirties*.

Common Pattern of Sustained Hypertension in Middle-Aged Adults

Adult hypertensives have *high peripheral vascular resistance.* Vessels have thick walls, but may not yet be atherosclerotic. The changes are presumably reversible at this stage (e.g., at about 35 to 45 years of age.) Arteries in adult hypertensives are hyperresponsive to pressor substances such as norepinephrine. It is unknown whether this hypersensitivity is the basic lesion of hypertension or is the result of hypertrophied vascular smooth muscle.

Adult patients with hypertension at mid-life have normal or even low cardiac output.

In established hypertension there is *low plasma volume.* The higher the pressure, the lower the plasma volume.

In established hypertension, the *kidneys* have subtle abnormalities, including excessive atherosclerosis and increased renal vascular resistance.

Pressure rises through adulthood as a function of the pressure earlier in life. In other words, those with pressures at age 30 that are slightly above average have pressures at 40 that are even higher above average. Put another way, the rise of pressure with age is faster for hypertensives than for normals.

The population as a whole contains a large group of normotensives whose pressure *never* rises and a smaller group of hypertensives whose pressure rises progressively with time. This may account for the finding that a whole population's average pressure tends to rise with age. In other words, *it is not inevitable that a normal individual's pressure rises with age.*

Much (but not all) of the rise of pressure with age can be attributed to the rise of *weight* with age.

In many people, the rise in pressure experienced beyond age 65 is primarily systolic, and caused by atherosclerosis. ''Stiff pipes'' are noncompliant, so the blood ejected by the heart is driven straight to the periphery without any buffering of the pressure wave by the aorta. During diastole, there is no rebound from the aorta, so peripheral pressure drops sharply. This causes a wide spread between systolic and diastolic readings, a wide ''pulse pressure.''

Evolution from First to Second Stage

A popular theory is that pressure, sporadically raised by the heart's response to high catecholamines, stress, etc., leads to thickened vessels in the periphery, including those in the kidney. The thick-walled vessels raise peripheral resistance. The thick renal vessels reduce the kidneys' ability to excrete salt or stimulate their output of renin. This can be thought of as an *inciting* cause in the *CNS* leading to a *sustaining* cause in *peripheral* vessels.

Another construction of the evolution of hypertension envisions an initial preponderance of β-adrenergic activity (high cardiac output) followed by a later preponderance of α-adrenergic activity (high peripheral resistance). How this shift might occur is not explained.

Stage of Complications

Complications occur earlier the higher the pressure.

In late hypertension, arteries are atherosclerotic. This is visible in the retina as ''increased light reflex,'' ''copper-wire,'' and ''silver-wire'' arteries. Some of these changes are irreversible (e.g., calcified vessels).

The heart is hypertrophic.

Small aneurysms exist in cerebral vessels (''Charcot-Bouchard'' aneurysms).

Kidney function is clearly decreased.

It is common to find pure *systolic hypertension* in older people with atherosclerosis. Pure systolic hypertension is dangerous in and of itself. It is especially dangerous to arteries of the brain and to the aorta. Systolic hypertension is also hard on the heart, which must generate the systolic pressure in order to eject blood. The old idea that diastolic or mean pressures are the only relevant parameters for morbid events is wrong. Pure systolic hypertension can kill.

As mentioned above, there is an epidemiologic pattern of *susceptibility to complications* that is distinct from susceptibility to hypertension. Blacks suffer more from a given pressure level than whites do, Japanese get strokes whereas Westerners get coronaries, etc. The basis for this pattern is almost surely genetic, but its mechanism is unknown. Family history is the only reasonable guide to the clinician who tries to predict the fate of his/her patients.

Subgroups of Essential Hypertension

Low-Renin Essential Hypertension (LREH)

One-fourth to one-third of all hypertensives have a *low* plasma renin activity, which responds sluggishly to standard stimuli such as upright posture or diuretics. Is it not ironic that while we search for pressor chemicals that can raise pressure, the most common chemical abnormality in all hypertensives is an unusually *low* level of the famous pressor renin!?

Despite the low plasma renin (and angiotensin) activity in LREH, plasma aldosterone and aldosterone excretion are *normal*. This condition may reflect super-sensitive adrenal glands (requiring less angiotensin for equal steroidogenesis), the presence of another stimulus to aldosterone, or an unrecognized mineralocorticoid that suppresses renin.

Patients with LREH have a faster-than-normal excretion of an acute sodium load. It looks like they are over-filled with fluid, and any extra load spills over. This is called "exaggerated natriuresis."

This condition should be differentiated from primary aldosteronism, and from the combination of *low-renin and low-aldosterone* levels when renin release is impaired by diabetes or dysautonomia.

Hyperdynamic (Hyperkinetic) Hypertension

This is characterized by rapid pulse and increased cardiac output. It is hard to dissociate from the early stage of essential hypertension and from pheochromocytoma.

This condition is almost certainly caused by excess β-adrenergic activity.

Summary

Essential hypertension, like the common cold and cancer, is extremely widespread and very mysterious. We know who gets it but we do not know why.

Hypertension at different stages of pathogenesis constitutes a spectrum of cardiovascular changes ranging from high cardiac output with low resistance to low cardiac output with sclerotic vessels and high peripheral resistance.

The most recent break in the monolith of essential hypertension is the classification by plasma renin levels. Low Renin Essential Hypertension (LREH) is probably a separate type of hypertension, resembling hyperaldosteronism in many ways.

11

Pathology of Hypertension*

Introduction

There are two aspects to the pathology associated with hypertension: the pathology of conditions *causing* hypertension and the pathologic *effects* of hypertension. This chapter focuses on the latter.

The *pathologic effects of hypertension* can be summarized as follows:

1. The pathologic effects of prolonged systemic hypertension are primarily reflected in the vascular system.

*This chapter was written with Dr. Enid Gilbert.

2. Hypertension is one of the major "risk factors" in the development of arteriosclerosis. (The other major factors are smoking, high blood lipids, and genetic predisposition.)
3. The target organs most commonly damaged by hypertension are the *aorta and its branches, heart, kidneys, brain,* and *retina.*
4. Hypertension and cancer are two common diseases wherein the body makes too much of something. In hypertension, the vessels and heart synthesize more of themselves, leading to *hyperplasia and hypertrophy that impairs function.* In the following paragraphs, note how many descriptive terms indicate excessive amounts of tissue.

Effects of Hypertension on the Arteries

Large Arteries

Atherosclerosis is accelerated by hypertension, particularly in the aorta and its major branches, most importantly in the coronary and cerebral vessels. In the larger arteries and branches of the aorta, elastic hyperplasia with reduplication of the internal elastic lamella occurs. *In general, the amount of elastic tissue in the wall of an artery reflects the blood pressure to which it has been exposed* (Fig. 1).

Small Arteries and Arterioles

The hallmarks of the vascular effects of hypertension are lesions of the small arteries and arterioles. These changes can be described as follows:

Hyperplastic Arteriolosclerosis

This is the most common lesion in hypertension. It begins with hypertrophy of the smooth muscle in the medial layer.

Medial hypertrophy may progress to *subintimal fibrosis* and *hyalinization* which may involve the entire wall of the vessel, and ultimately obliterate the lumen.

Smooth muscle proliferation also occurs in the intima. The sum of all changes can lead to a condition called "onion skinning," caused by concentric reduplication and lamination of elastic layers and smooth muscle fibers (Fig. 2).

The pathogenetic sequence in the development of hyperplastic arteriolosclerosis is as follows:

1. Breaks occur in the elastic lamella, allowing migration of smooth muscle fibers into the intima.
2. Breaks occur in the endothelium, allowing sticking of platelets and the

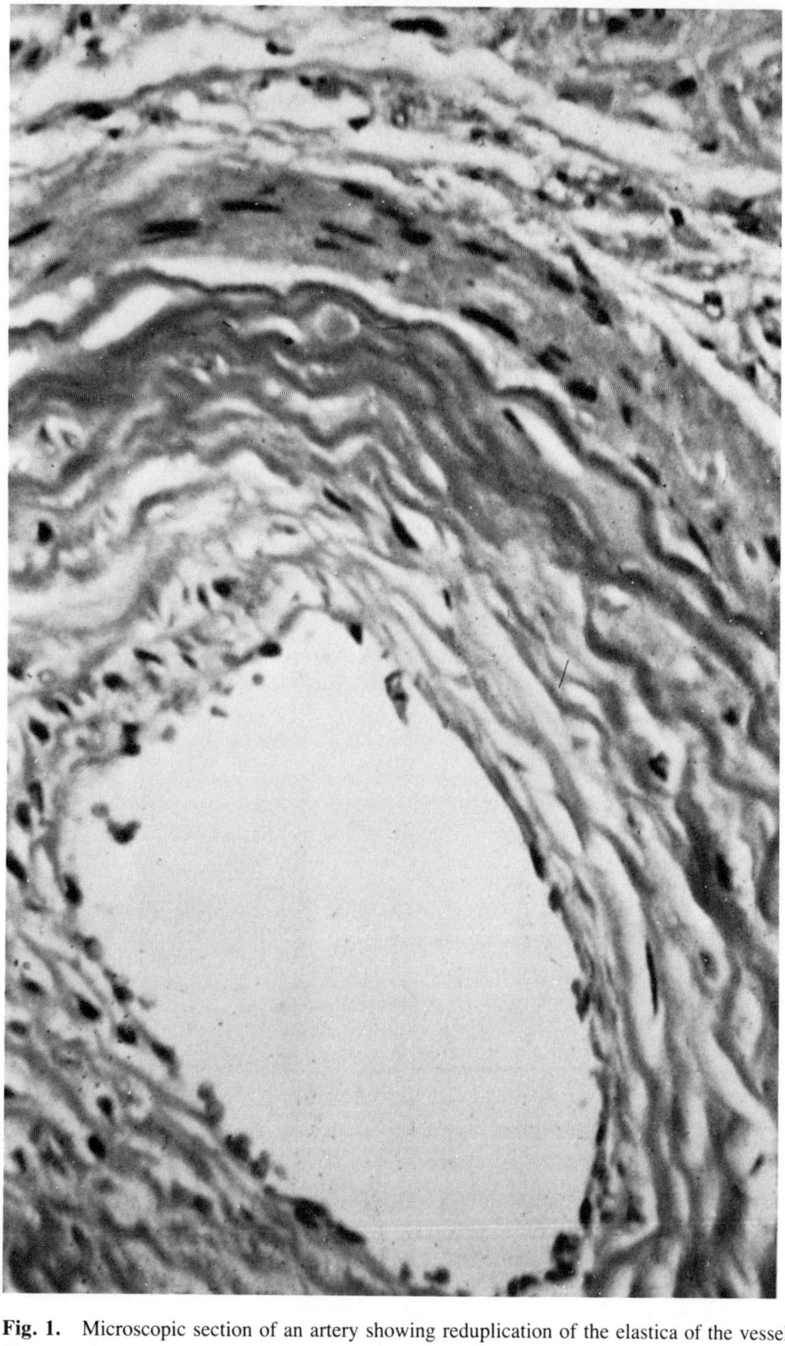

Fig. 1. Microscopic section of an artery showing reduplication of the elastica of the vessel wall as seen in hypertension. (H & E stain. Mag. ×100.)

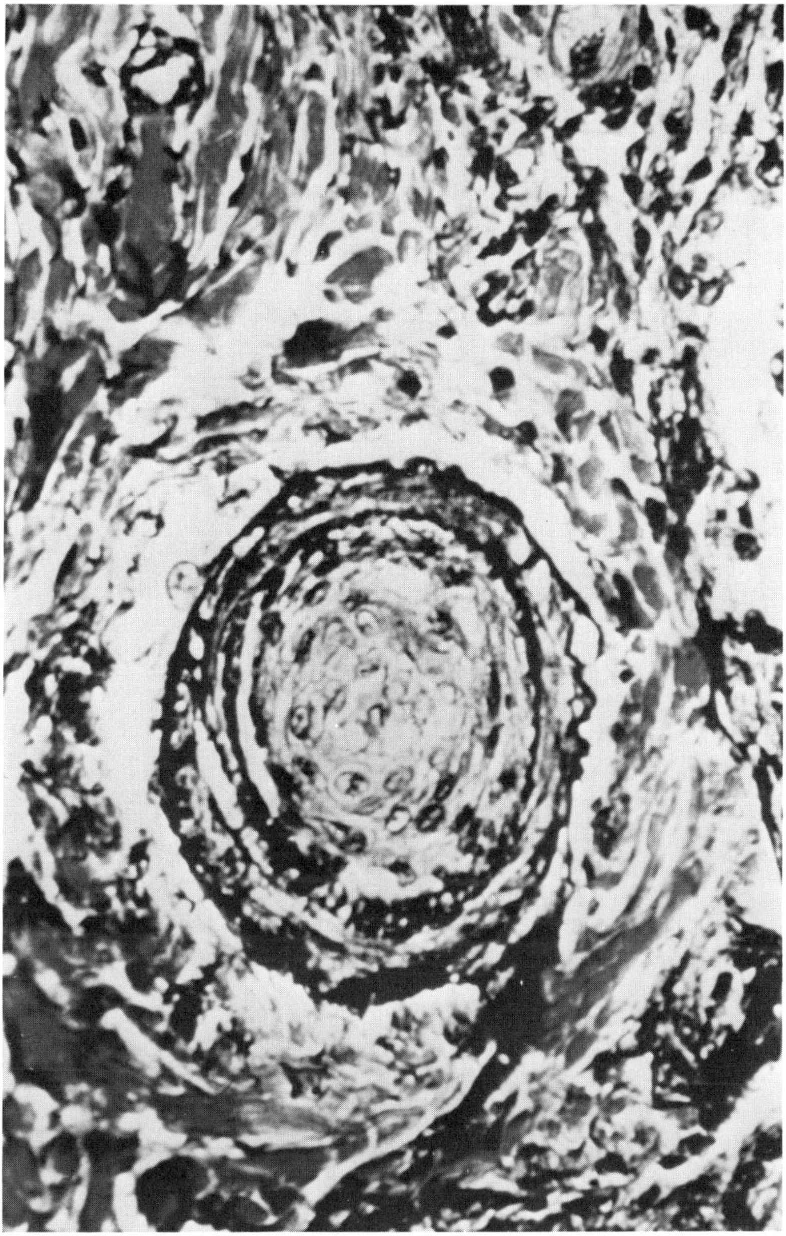

Fig. 2. Microscopic section of small vessel showing hyperplastic arteriolitis. The media is thickened and there is intimal proliferation with almost complete obliteration of the lumen. (Elastic Van Gieson stain. Mag. ×100.)

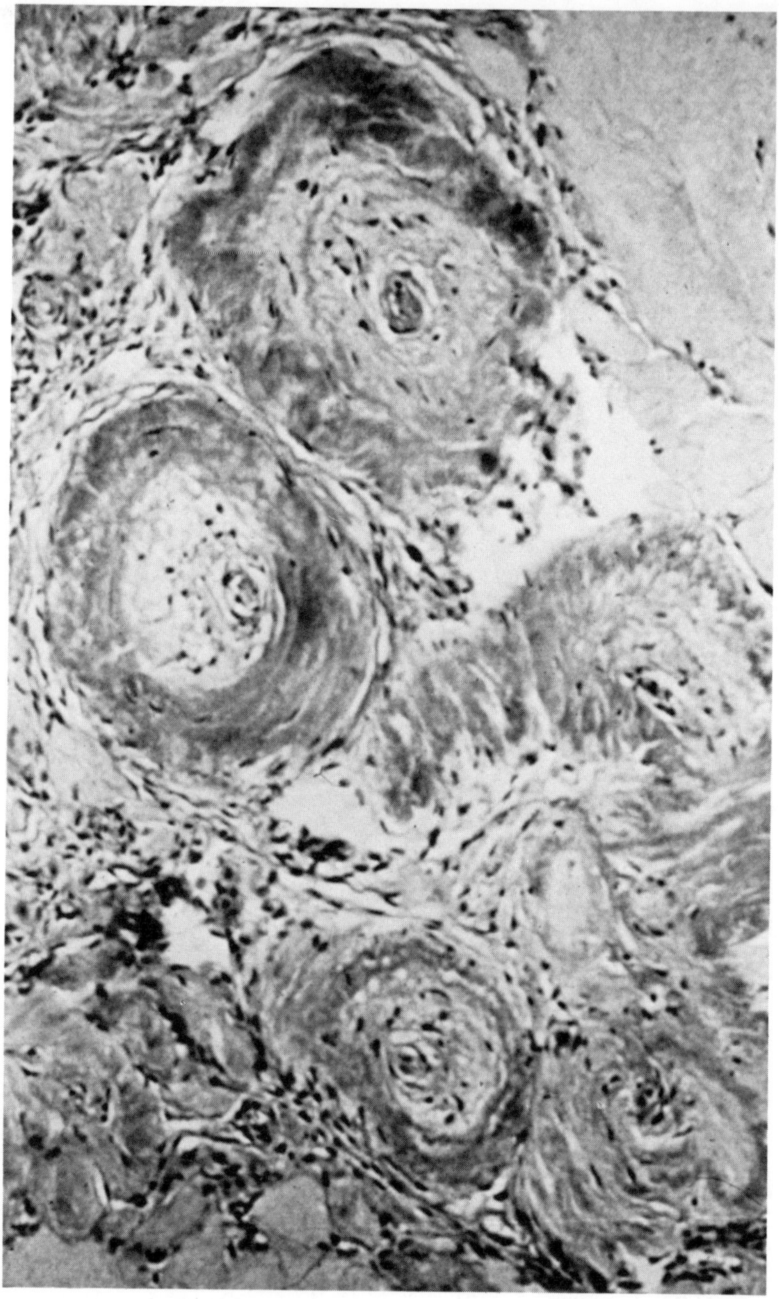

Fig. 3. Microscopic section of several small arteries showing thick hyalinized walls "hyaline sclerosis." (H & E stain. Mag. ×100.)

entrance of lipids, factors that stimulate smooth muscle cell growth, and other material from the blood that may initiate the atherosclerotic process. These breaks may be caused in part by effects of pressors such as angiotensin, which can cause endothelial cells to contract and separate from one another, leaving "interendothelial gaps."

3. Medial muscle fibers hypertrophy and the elastic lamella reduplicates.

Hyaline Sclerosis

Hyaline sclerosis involves the intima and media (Fig. 3). The intimal elastic lamella becomes thickened and frayed in this condition. This is a common lesion, not solely a result of hypertension. On electron microscopic examination, "hyaline" proves to be thickened basement membrane made mostly of collagen.

Hyaline sclerosis is most prominent in interlobular and afferent glomerular arterioles of the kidney.

In some elderly, normotensive individuals, hyaline sclerosis lesions may occur which are indistinguishable from the lesions of hypertension. In these instances, it may be impossible to tell whether the lesions are consequences of hypertension or of degenerative changes related to age.

Aneurysms

Hypertension predisposes to *arteriosclerotic* aneurysms.

Hypertension potentiates the aortic lesion of cystic medionecrosis, the precursor of *dissecting* aortic aneurysms, and contributes to the rupture (dissection) of the vessel's inner layers.

Hypertension predisposes to rupture of cerebral *berry* aneurysms in the Circle of Willis. Hypertension does not cause these, but it does promote their rupture (Fig. 4).

Hypertension causes *microaneurysms* in small cerebral arteries within the brain ("Charcot-Bouchard aneurysms"). They are characteristic of hypertension (see below).

The development and rupture of aneurysms is particularly related to high *systolic* pressures.

The Heart

Gross Anatomy

Concentric left ventricular hypertrophy is the classical change in the heart with hypertension. Hypertrophy is manifested by thickening of the left ventricular myocardium (normal thickness up to about 1.2 cm) without enlargement of the ventricular chamber (Fig. 5). On chest X ray, the heart size is seen

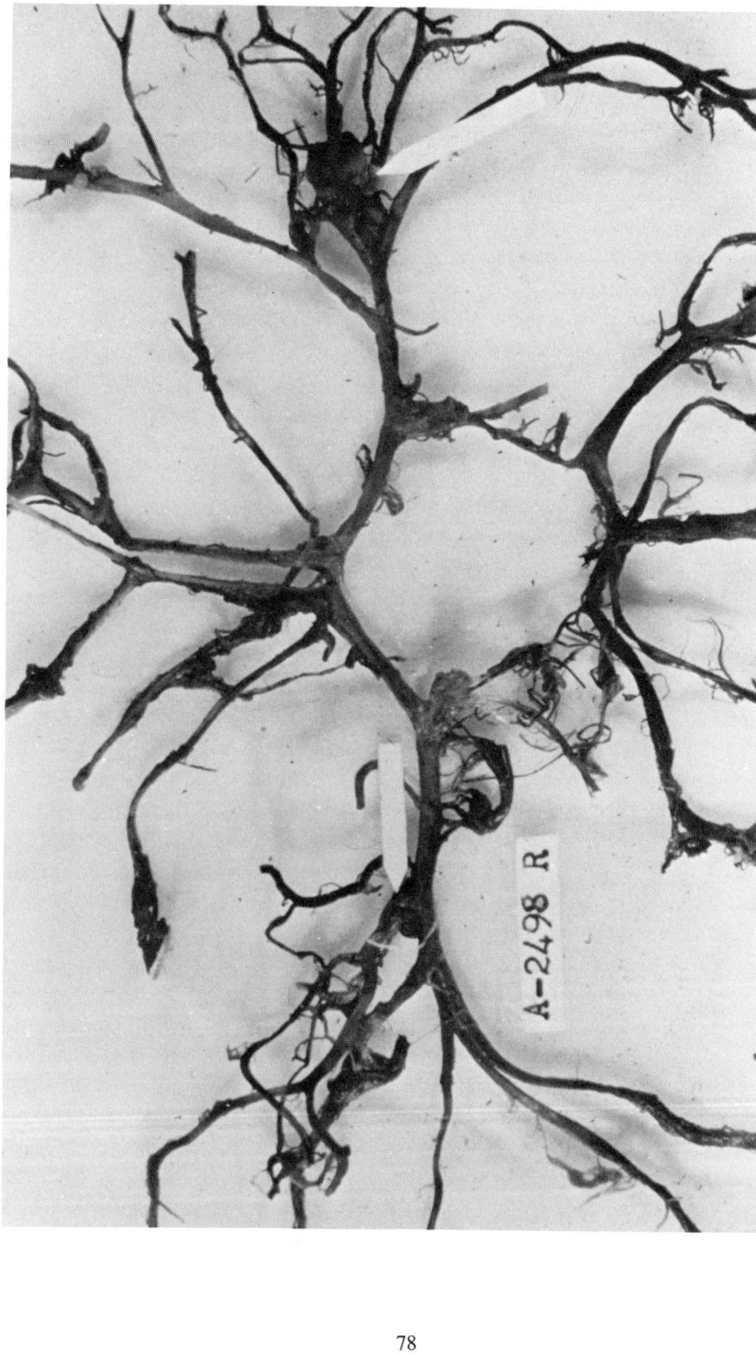

Fig. 4. Vessels at the base of the brain showing multiple berry aneurysms at branching points of the Circle of Willis—a common source of subarachnoid hemorrhage in hypertension.

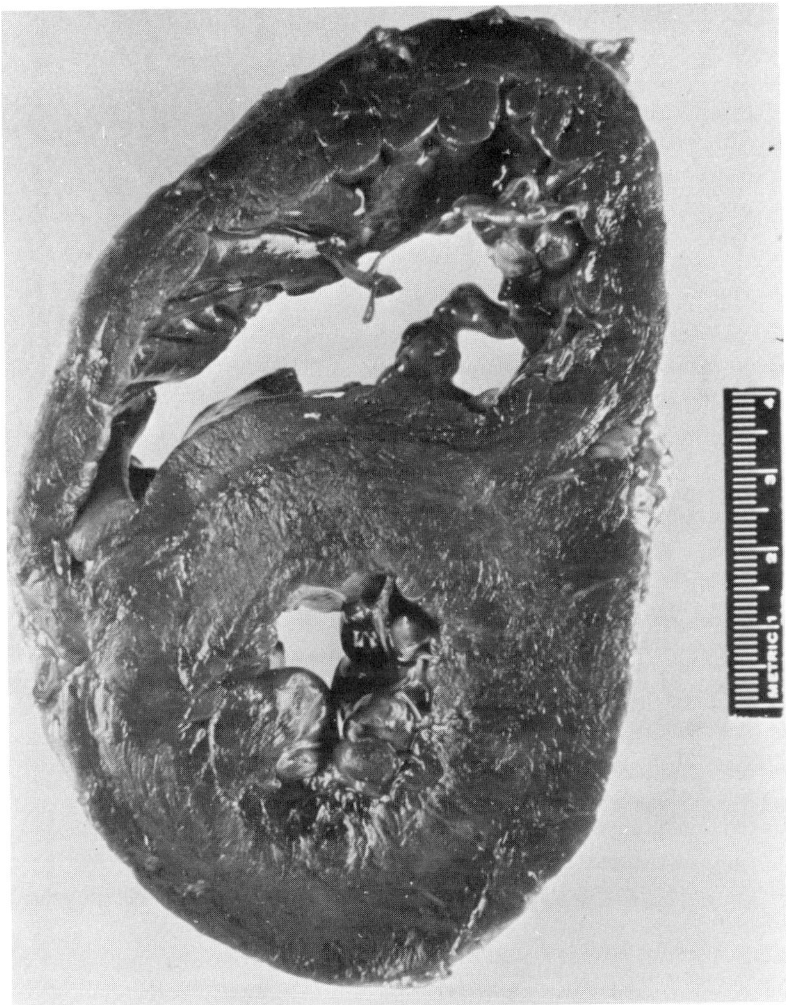

Fig. 5. Cross-section of the heart showing marked myocardial hypertrophy in hypertension.

to be normal at the stage of concentric hypertrophy, but the electrocardiogram shows increased voltage changes with each beat, because of the increased mass of myocardium.

In the absence of other cardiac lesions, heart weight reflects the degree of left ventricular hypertrophy. Normally, the heart weight is 0.40–0.45% of total body weight. (This proportion is lower in obese individuals and is slightly lower in women than men.) For practical purposes, the normal upper limit of heart weight is 350–375 gm for women and 375–400 gm for men.

Physiological hypertrophy can occur as a result of prolonged physical exercise, with the heart weight reaching 500 gm ("critical heart weight"). In physiologic hypertrophy, myocardial fibers lengthen and thicken.

Once "critical heart weight" is exceeded, hyperplasia occurs (increase in the number of individual cells). The heart weight of patients who succumb to hypertensive heart disease and its usual complications is commonly in the neighborhood of 500–700 gm. In extreme instances of long-standing severe hypertension, heart weight may reach 1000 gm or more. Hearts that are heavier than 700–800 gm are termed "*cor bovinum,*" because they resemble in size the hearts of cattle.

The relationship between muscle fibers and capillaries remains constant during *physiological* hypertrophy (i.e., there is a proportional increase in capillaries). When critical heart size is exceeded, as in hypertension, the increased demand for oxygen is not met by capillary growth, and foci of ischemic necrosis may develop, leading eventually to focal scarring (fibrosis).

Microscopic Changes

In hypertrophy, the diameter of myocardial fibers is thickened to as much as 20 μm (normal 5–12 μm) by increased sarcoplasm and myofibrils.

Nuclei are hyperchromatic and rectangular ("box-car nuclei").

Degenerative changes, such as vacuolization of the fibers, increased pigment (lipofuscin), and basophilia of the sarcoplasm, may occur.

There is an increase in enzyme systems that can be demonstrated histochemically.

Ultrastructural changes of hypertrophy include: increase in the number of mitochondria, enlargement of sarcoplasmic tubules, accumulation of glycogen, prominence of the Golgi apparatus, increase in number of myofibrils, and widening of the "Z band."

Complications Involving the Heart

Left ventricular failure is a common complication of hypertension. When failure occurs, the left ventricle dilates and then may show "eccentric" hypertrophy. Left ventricular failure is clearly made more likely by the presence of hypertension. The chest X ray in a case with the combination of failure and hypertrophy shows an enlarged cardiac silhouette.

Hypertensive heart disease may be the underlying condition in some cases of unexplained *cardiomyopathy,* with or without heart failure. Confusion arises when the hypertensive heart fails and pressure falls. (This is a frequent event after myocardial infarction.) The patient may have a heart that looks hypertrophic; but the cause of hypertrophy is obscure because blood pressure is low, so the term "idiopathic cardiomyopathy" is applied. Many patients with hypertrophic hearts and normal blood pressure are actually in the final stages of hypertensive heart disease.

Increased arterial pressure leads to more rapid atherosclerosis of the coronary arteries and *myocardial infarction*. At least two-thirds of all myocardial infarcts are in patients with hypertension. Hypertension is the best-identified risk factor for myocardial infarction.

Hypertension also aggravates the *poor function* of a diseased heart. By demanding more work, high arterial pressure drives the heart to consume more oxygen and nutrients, and may induce heart failure if the coronary circulation is diminished or the myocardium diseased. "Pressure work" is more demanding on the heart than "output work," so high arterial pressure is the ultimate stress on a diseased heart. The mechanism whereby pressure work makes unusual demands is unknown.

The Kidney

Hypertension causes the lesions collectively known as *arteriolar nephrosclerosis*.

1. These renal lesions include *hyperplastic arteriolosclerosis* and *hyaline sclerosis* of the arterioles.
2. In addition, the larger interlobular and arcuate arteries exhibit a characteristic lesion called *fibroelastic hyperplasia*. This is marked by reduplication of the elastic lamina and increased fibrous tissue in the *media,* with consequent narrowing of the lumen.
3. Grossly, the kidneys with nephrosclerosis have a "cobblestone" appearance—uniformly granular—caused by multiple areas of fibrotic scars between areas of healthy tissue.

The kidney in *malignant hypertension* evolves as follows:

1. Malignant hypertension (defined as a rapidly increasing pressure) causes the appearance of small pinpoint petechial hemorrhages on the

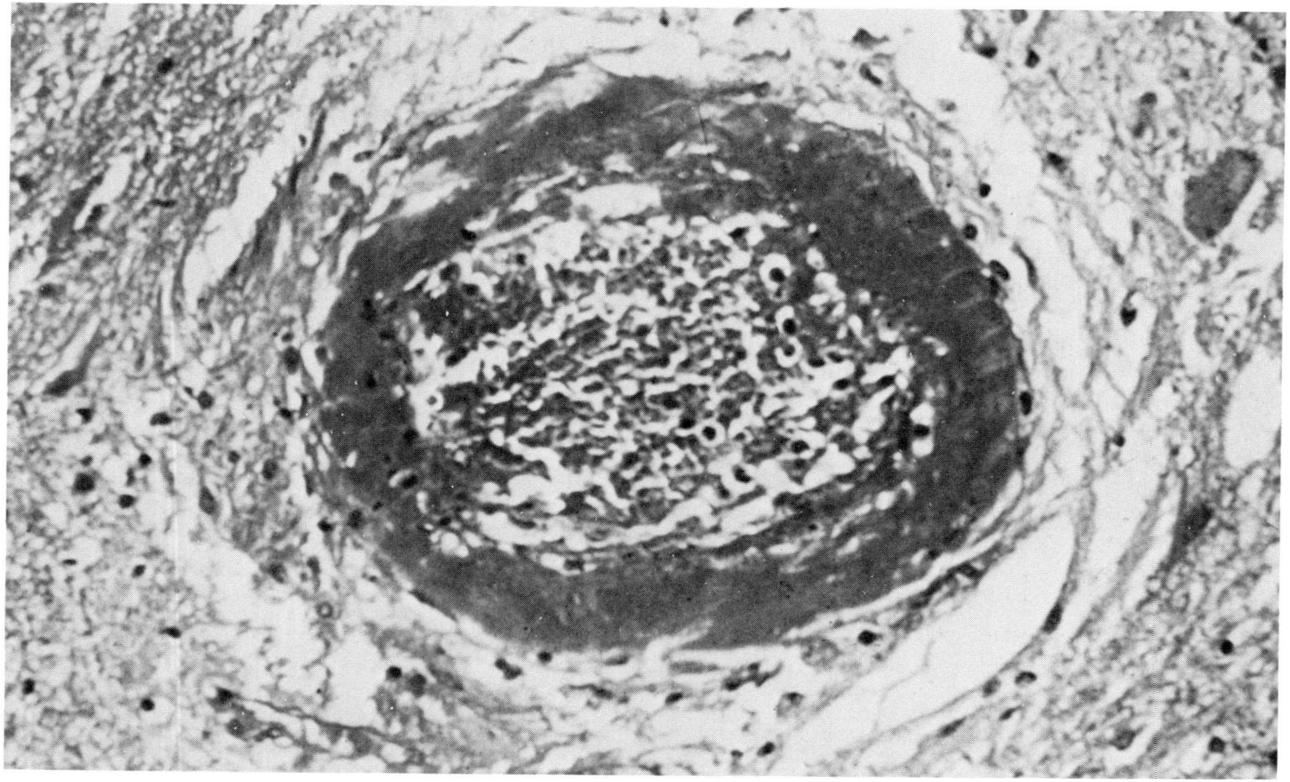

Fig. 6. Microscopic section of arteriole in malignant hypertension showing necrotizing arteriolitis with fibrinoid change of vessel wall. (H & E stain. Mag. ×100.)

cortical surface of the kidneys, from rupture of arterioles or glomerular capillaries. This gives the kidney a peculiar "flea-bitten" appearance.

2. Several histologic alterations characterize malignant hypertension.
   a. *Fibrinoid necrosis* of arterioles (Fig. 6) appears as an eosinophilic granular change in the blood vessel wall, which stains positively for fibrin by histochemical or immunofluorescent techniques. The fibrin can replace cellular elements of the vessel wall. Fibrinoid changes occur when rupture of elastic lamellae leads to excessive exudate of clotting factors from plasma that then organize in the vessel wall.
   b. In addition, there is often an *inflammatory* infiltrate within the walls of renal vessels, giving rise to the term *necrotizing arteriolitis*. This change can occur elsewhere in the body in malignant hypertension.
   c. In the larger interlobular arteries, there is a characteristic *intimal* thickening caused by a proliferation of elongated, concentrically arranged smooth muscle cells, together with fine concentric layering of collagen. This alteration is known as *hyperplastic arteriolitis*. (It differs from the hyperplastic arterio*sclerosis* of ordinary hypertension in its tendency to have an inflammatory component.)
   d. Glomeruli may thrombose in malignant hypertension. This is called *necrotizing glomerulitis*. If these necrotic capillaries rupture, they cause hemorrhages into the glomerular spaces and adjacent tubules, causing the flea-bitten appearance mentioned above.
   e. The arteriolar and arterial lesions result in considerable narrowing of all vascular lumina, with ischemia and *infarctions* distal to the abnormal vessels.

The question of *cause* and *effect* enters into all discussions of renal pathology in hypertension.

1. Clearly, renal vessels are damaged as an *effect* of hypertension.
2. The nature of the vascular damage is such that arteries develop smaller lumens. Smaller arterial lumens are the *cause of renovascular hypertension* (either by stimulating release of renin or by reducing sodium excretion).
3. It is generally accepted that the kidneys participate in a *vicious cycle*, with renal vascular damage resulting from hypertension, and renal vascular insufficiency causing persistent hypertension.
4. The ability of damaged kidneys to *perpetuate* hypertension (even when they were not the original cause) accounts for most failures when

curable causes are corrected too late. Thus, removal of a tumor secreting aldosterone may be curative only 70% of the time, because the hypertension caused by the tumor had already damaged the kidneys and they perpetuate hypertension after tumor removal.

The Brain

Strokes

Hypertension predisposes to *strokes* (cerebrovascular accidents or "CVAs") in several ways:

1. Accelerated atherosclerosis, with thrombosis of large arteries causing brain infarction. The intimal plaques and narrowing of lumen predispose to thrombi. This hypertension-associated sclerosis accounts for 80% of all strokes.
2. Rupture of berry aneurysms of the Circle of Willis, with subarachnoid hemorrhage. This accounts for another 10% of all strokes.
3. Rupture of tiny microaneurysms in the small cerebral vessels ("Charcot–Bouchard aneurysms") with hemorrhage into the brain parenchyma. This accounts for the final 10% of all strokes.

Charcot–Bouchard Aneurysms

Development of these tiny aneurysms appears to be directly related to arterial pressure. These lesions occur principally in small perforating arteries of less than 1-mm diameter, especially in the basal ganglia and cortical regions (lenticulo-striate vessels). They are characterized by loss of the media (the intima and adventitia are unaffected). The wall of the vessel is thus weakened and becomes aneurysmal. Under high arterial pressure, rupture may occur with massive intracerebral hemorrhage, far out of proportion to the size of the aneurysm (Fig. 7).

Lacunae

A change resembling swiss cheese can be seen in cut sections of the brain in hypertensives. After infarction caused by occlusion of small vessels, the cells of the infarcted brain die, and cysts are left behind.

Transient Ischemic Attacks (TIAs)

These are episodes of transient focal cerebral ischemia, causing transient loss of some cerebral functions. This is a clinical condition with no charac-

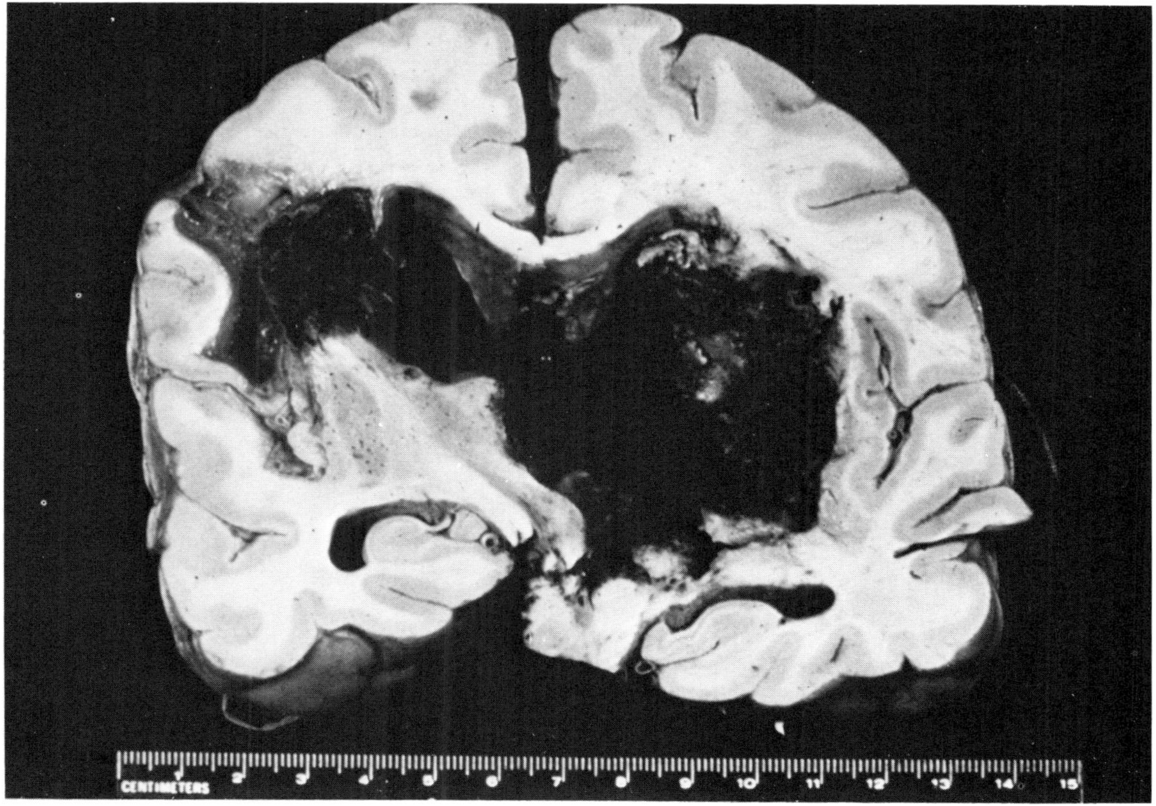

Fig. 7. Coronal section of the brain showing massive hemorrhage and destruction of the brain substance due to rupture of a Charcot–Bouchard aneurysm.

teristic pathologic lesion except atherosclerosis. Clinically, TIAs are marked by brief episodes of loss of consciousness, loss of speech, blindness or other visual change, confusion, dizziness, or paresthesias. TIAs are probably caused by microemboli from arteriosclerotic plaques or by platelet pile-ups in narrowed vessels. Hypertension aggravates TIAs, probably because it damages endothelium, causing platelet adhesion, causes temporary arterial spasm and narrowing, or simply aggravates and accelerates atherosclerosis.

The Retina

Microscopic sections of arterioles of the retina in hypertension show several changes, most of which are actually atherosclerotic in nature and not pathognomonic for hypertension. These include:

1. *Thickening* of arterial wall. During life, the hypertensive's retina displays apparent *narrowing* of arterioles in the retina. This is an illusion, because we only visualize the column of blood in the vessel and not the vessel wall. The vessel as a whole is actually thickened in hypertension. In addition, these thick-walled arteries press on the soft veins where they criss-cross. This causes the well-known "A-V nicking" or "crossing defects" seen on examination of the retina during life.
2. *Hemorrhages* into the retina result from ruptured arterioles in severe hypertension.
3. *Exudates,* composed of partially reabsorbed hemorrhages, can be seen pre- and postmortem in the retina of some hypertensive patients. They can be cottony or waxy in gross appearance.

The pathognomonic retinal sign of hypertension seen during life is *arteriolar spasm* (segmental narrowing). This is not seen postmortem because the vessels relax after death.

In malignant hypertension, there is edema of the retina and of the optic nerve, leading finally to papilledema.

Cause of Death

The cause of death in hypertensives breaks down statistically as follows:

1. Congestive heart failure: 45% (Hypertension is a causative factor in 75% of all cases of congestive heart failure.)
2. Coronary insufficiency or myocardial infarction: 35%
3. Cerebral vascular accident: 15%
4. Renal failure: 5%

Summary

Early pathologic changes caused by hypertension reflect synthetic activities in the heart and vessels, and are marked by hyperplasia and thickening. Atherosclerosis is accelerated by hypertension.

Later pathological changes in hypertension are marked by the scars following infarctions in the brain, heart, and kidneys.

The most dramatic events induced by hypertension are sudden ruptures or occlusions of arteries in the head and heart.

12 Diagnostic Evaluation of Patients with Hypertension

Introduction

Every patient with hypertension must be evaluated with respect to four considerations (to help your memory, use the acronym *PEET: P*ressure, *E*tiology, *E*ffects, *T*herapy):

1. The level of the blood *pressure* itself
2. The *etiology* of the pressure elevation
3. *Effects* the high pressure has already exerted on target organs
4. Aspects of the patient that might affect choices of *therapy*

Measuring the Pressure

The common methods are all indirect, using a cuff around the arm, a manometer to measure pressure in the cuff, and a stethoscope or other device to detect pulsations in an artery distal to the cuff. The manometer records the pressure of air in a rubber bladder or balloon in the cuff, which in turn presses on flesh, which in turn presses on an artery, whose flow is heard downstream. The observer inflates the cuff-balloon, watches the pressure in it, and listens for sounds in the distal vessel as the balloon is deflated. The manometer does *not* record pressure in the artery, but the assumption is made that the pressure in the cuff-balloon is equal to the pressure at the wall of the artery. Artifacts are created when the pressure in the balloon is inefficiently transmitted to the artery wall.

The most important factor in obtaining an accurate pressure reading is the size of the cuff and its contained air bladder. *The cuff must be large enough.* The most common error in pressure recording is the use of a cuff that is too small. A small cuff reads the pressure too high. Many a fat person has been miraculously "cured" of hypertension by the sudden use of a larger cuff! (This error is almost inexcusable.) The general idea is to use a cuff whose entire head of air pressure will be directed inward toward the artery, and not wasted squeezing laterally on fat or inefficiently trapped under a narrow wrapper.

1. The width of the cuff must be at least two-thirds the length of the upper arm.
2. The inflatable balloon or bladder should be long enough to encircle two thirds of the arm's circumference.
3. In case of large, fatty, or muscular arms, either use an extra-large cuff, or wrap the cuff around the *fore*arm, and detect the pulse at the *wrist.*
4. The cuff *can* be too large, but only in cases where huge cuffs are used on tiny arms. If the bladder wraps around upon itself, part of the pressure in it is used to press on the underlying bladder, not on the flesh of the arm.

The manometer must be calibrated regularly. (This is especially true of aneroid dials.) Periodically, use a Y tube and record bladder pressure with the aneroid dial and a mercury manometer at the same time. Do not use a dial that has a "peg" to which the needle returns. This makes it impossible to tell if the zero reading has shifted.

Inflate the cuff rapidly, within 15 sec, to avoid filling the arm with venous blood while the cuff is below arterial pressure. An engorged arm is harder to compress than a flaccid one.

Avoid the "auscultatory gap" by *palpating* the pulse during inflation. This is a problem in only a minority of patients. The "auscultatory gap" is a region of pressure between systolic and diastolic where Korotkoff sounds are not heard. If *initial* cuff pressure falls in that gap, systolic pressures will be read too low. If you inflate the cuff only to a level within the gap, the first sound is heard far below true systolic pressure. (Some aspects of measurement and its problems are illustrated in Fig. 1.)

Deflate the cuff 2–3 mm per sec. Do not let the patient watch the indicator. They *all* think their pressures are indicated by the bouncing that begins to show in the mercury or dial at pressures well above systolic. (The bouncing is irrelevant.)

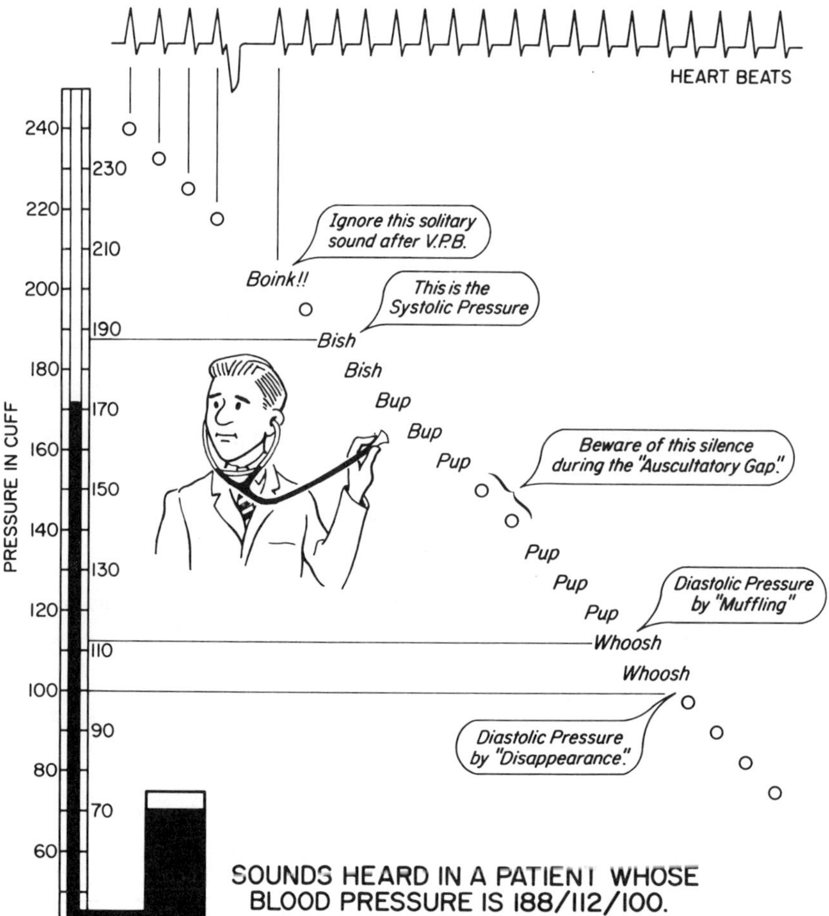

Fig. 1. Schematic example of the measurement of arterial blood pressure in a patient with one ventricular premature beat (VPB), causing a single high-pressure pulse thereafter, and a silent auscultatory gap of unknown cause (and no significance). Avoiding these distractions, the observer calmly notes the first Korotkoff sound of a regular series, the first muffled beat, and the point at which silence begins. He records all three.

Read exact pressures. *Do not round-off* to the nearest multiple of 5. If you deflate slowly enough, you can read smaller intervals.

Systolic pressure is that pressure below which a tap is heard at *each beat* (not just with extra systoles or during forced expiration).

The diastolic pressure is the point of *disappearance* of sounds (Phase V).

1. If *disappearance* (Phase V) is widely different from *muffling* (Phase IV), record both (e.g., "140/80/60"). This is a universally recognized notation.
2. Disappearance is used as the customary indicator because it is more reliable from observer to observer. Different people recognize "muffling" as different sounds.
3. In some patients, especially children with high flows through small vessels, disappearance of sounds occurs much lower than muffling. In fact, some people have Korotkoff sounds over their artery with no cuff at all. *In those people, the muffling is probably a better indication of the true diastolic pressure.*

Wait 2 min with the cuff fully deflated before repeating. This avoids artifacts caused by venous filling while the cuff is above venous pressure.

Measure *both arms* and *one thigh* at the first visit.

1. Sometimes, kinking or atherosclerosis of branches from the aorta cause falsely low pressure in one arm.
2. Use the *higher* of the two arm pressures to guide therapy and prognosis. Write down which arm you measured.
3. Thigh pressure is taken only once to rule out coarctation. Apply a large cuff around the thigh and listen in the popliteal fossa, with the patient supine.

Measure pressure supine and upright (after 2 min standing) as well as sitting. Record the *position* of the patient, as well as the *limb* measured, and *Phase IV/Phase V* readings. This is to serve as baseline for a possible side effect of treatment, "postural hypotension." Although most people show no significant difference upon standing, 20% of the elderly have a significant pressure drop even before therapy has been started.

Repeat pressure at *three visits* before deciding on therapy, unless the pressure is clearly and dangerously elevated. Patient fear or anxiety almost always causes higher pressure at the first visit. The more forebidding you appear, or the harder it is to park near your office, the higher the "initial visit artifact." The natural tendency for pressure to fall to normal after several visits (when patients learn where to park, etc.) could be improperly interpreted as pharmacologic success if drugs were begun immediately.

Special tricks for measuring pressure in infants include using the "skin flush," a Doppler probe, or a second cuff as indicators when Korotkoff sounds cannot be heard.

1. To use the "skin flush," first squeeze the blood out of the *lower* arm by wrapping it tightly with an ace bandage; then apply the blood pressure cuff to the *upper* arm, and inflate; then remove the wrap from the forearm and watch for pinking of the skin as the cuff is deflated to systolic pressure. (Only systolic pressure is read by this method.)
2. A Doppler flow probe can be used in place of the stethoscope to detect flow in the brachial artery as the cuff is deflated.
3. A second cuff below the first, inflated to about 30 mm, will show "bouncing" of its dial when the upper cuff falls below systolic pressure.

Some elderly patients with calcified vessels may have readings that are falsely elevated, because the balloon pressure needed to occlude a calcified tube is high even when the blood in the tube is under normal pressure. This is referred to as "pseudohypertension." When treated with hypotensive drugs, these patients experience *low* intravascular pressure, especially on standing. There is no way to avoid this, except by suspecting pseudohypertension when the pressures measured in different limbs are significantly different, maybe lower in the legs than the arms, with vessel calcification seen in X rays. (It may be reasonable to clear this up once and for all by a quick visit to the CCU where intraarterial pressure can be recorded directly.)

Etiology

All modalities of clinical evaluation are used to check for the existence of well-understood hypertension: the history, physical exam, lab, X ray, and others. Essential hypertension is diagnosed only by exclusion, when no identifiable causes are found. Remember RECAP, the mnemonic for curable causes: *R*enal, *E*strogens, *C*oarctation, *A*ldosteronism, and *P*heochromocytoma.

Identifiable (but not always curable) etiologies listed in decreasing order of frequency include:

1. Obesity
2. Birth-control pills containing estrogen
3. Renal diseases of all types
4. Alcohol abuse
5. Adrenal cortical hyperfunction, with mineralocorticoid excess

TABLE I

Clues from the History That Suggest Specific Causes of Hypertension

Cause	*Clue*
Obesity	Weight gain coincident with pressure rise
Estrogen-containing medication	Medication history. Note that many people do not think of their birth-control pills or nasal decongestant as "medication." Be *specific* in questioning (Be *subtle* with the suspected alcohol abuser.)
Renal diseases, including renal artery stenosis, glomerulonephritis, infection, familial polycystic disease, trauma, obstruction, or tumor	Burning on urination Frequent urination, nocturia Passage or stones or blood in urine Family history of renal disease Recent injury to flank, including surgery or X-ray therapy Pain in flank or groin
Adrenal cortical hyperfunction, including aldosteronoma	Weakness (from low K^+) Nocturia (from effect of low K^+ on renal concentrating mechanism)
Preeclampsia	Pregnancy history; edema
Pheochromocytoma	Episodes of Headache Sweating or flushing Palpitation Anxiety and tremor Nausea Family history of endocrine tumors, or pheochromocytomas
Coarctation of aorta	Leg pain on exercise "Heart murmur" heard by other physicians
Drugs that raise pressure	Ingestion of pressor drugs, such as nasal decongestants Ingestion of unusual amounts of licorice (!) Excessive alcohol intake (over 3 drinks per day)
General clues that suggest the presence of a specific, identifiable cause of hypertension	Onset of hypertension before 30 or after 50 Absence of family history of hypertension Abrupt onset or unusual magnitude of hypertension Failure of conventional therapy

6. Preeclampsia
7. Pheochromocytoma
8. Coarctation
9. Miscellaneous causes, such as drugs that raise pressure, hypothyroidism, hyperthyroidism, and hyperparathyroidism

General clues that tip off the clinician to the existence of an identifiable cause, as opposed to essential hypertension, include:

1. Onset of hypertension before 30 or after 50
2. Absence of a family history of hypertension

TABLE II

Clues from the Physical Exam that Suggest Specific Causes of Hypertension

Cause	*Clue*
Obesity	Obesity
Estrogen administration	Chloasma (facial pigment)
Renal diseases	
a. Renal artery stenosis	Bruit under ribs, anteriorly
b. Inflammation, infection, or trauma	Tender kidneys on deep palpation
c. Polycystic disease, obstruction, or tumor	Enlarged kidneys
Adrenal cortical hyperfunction	Aldosteronomas produce no signs, but evidence of *gluco*corticoid excess is seen when Cushing's Syndrome causes incidental hypertension.
Preeclampsia	Pregnancy
	Edema
Pheochromocytoma	Neurofibromas and Café-au-lait spots (can coexist with pheochromocytomas)
	Tumors of thyroid or parathyroid, or neuromas of lips in multiple endocrine adenomatosis
Coarctation of aorta	Pressure lower in leg than arm (especially after exercise)
	Palpable lag in pulse between neck and leg or foot
	Pulses palpable in intercostal spaces (from collaterals)
	Coexistent Turner's Syndrome, (gonadal dysgenesis in females)
Miscellaneous causes	
a. Hypothyroidism	Slow-pulse, speech, and reflexes
b. Hyperthyroidism	Fast everything

TABLE III

Clues from Routine Laboratory Tests and Routine X Rays That Suggest Specific Causes of Hypertension[a]

Cause	*Clue*
Obesity	None
Estrogen administration	None
Renal diseases	Any abnormality in urinalysis
	Elevated blood urea nitrogen (BUN) or serum creatinine
	Abnormal intravenous pyelogram (IVP)
Adrenal cortical hyperfunction	Low serum potassium (below 3.5 mEq/L)
	High blood glucose levels
Preeclampsia	Positive pregnancy test
	Protein in urine
Pheochromocytoma[a]	High blood glucose levels
Coarctation of aorta	Abnormal aortic shadow on chest X ray
	"Notching" of ribs on chest X ray, from collateral vessel hypertrophy
Miscellaneous causes	High serum calcium levels, suggesting hyperparathyroidism

[a] This list omits special tests designed to find specific causes (such as measurement of catecholamines, catheterization of renal vessels, etc.

3. Abrupt onset of hypertension (often suggested by the extremely high pressure seen at the first exam)
4. Poor response to initial therapy, or escape from control during therapy

Specific clues that suggest identifiable causes of hypertension are divided into history (Table I), physical exam (Table II), and lab and X ray (Table III), broken up according to the identifiable cause. These tables omit special tests that would be ordered only *after* suspicions about a specific disease had been aroused. To review the diagnostic picture of each separate cause, refer to the appropriate earlier sections.

Effects of Hypertension on Target Organs

Retinal Vessels

Examination of the retina (eyegrounds) is the best way to assess both hypertensive and atherosclerotic changes in vessels.

1. With the ophthalmoscope, look for *segmental narrowing* or *spasm* of the retinal arteries as signs of vasoconstriction. In its acute form, this narrowing looks like a string of sausages. Segmental narrowing is the

only true sign of hypertension itself and is the most rapidly reversible change during therapy. Generalized narrowing (resulting in an artery : vein ratio less than 2 : 3) is usually the combined result of atherosclerosis and hypertension. Narrowing alone, without other changes, places the retina in "Grade 1," according to a popular classification.

2. Look for "A-V nicking," also called "crossing defects." These are defects in the column of blood seen in *veins* as they course behind arterioles that are thick walled and under pressure. The veins look interrupted as they squeeze under the artery. *If these are seen more than one disk-diameter away from the optic disk* itself, they are signs of thick-walled arteries, usually caused by hypertension. (Crossing defects that occur very near the disk have NO significance.) This change takes years to develop. Spasm can occur in days or weeks. The presence of A-V nicking plus arteriolar narrowing places the retina in "Grade 2."
3. Look for hemorrhages or exudates, signs of severe structural damage to vessels. The hemorrhages caused by hypertension are flame-shaped, or linear, near the disk and its vessels. (Hemorrhages that are rounder or peripheral are more likely caused by diabetic microangiopathy.) Exudates can be yellow or white patches with clear ("hard") margins or fuzzy ("soft") margins. Hemorrhages or exudates put the retina in "Grade 3."
4. Papilledema, edema of the optic disk, is the most fearsome change in the hypertensive retina. It drops the retina into "Grade 4," and reflects a dire prognosis.
5. Other changes, such as increased reflectiveness of vessels ("silver-wiring" or "copper-wiring"), are difficult to quantify. They indicate atherosclerosis, not hypertension per se.
6. Acute changes in the retina include segmental (spastic) narrowing, hemorrhages, and papilledema. They can be reversed more readily than other changes. Chronic changes include generalized narrowing (which may be purely atherosclerotic), A-V nicking, and exudates (old hemorrhages). They reverse slowly.
7. The retina is the harbinger and historian of hypertension. It predicts how well the vessels (and the patient) will withstand elevated pressure, and it shows how much damage has already been done.

Peripheral Vessels

1. There may be a history of claudication (pain in the calves after walking a certain distance).
2. Examination may reveal reduced pulses to palpation and bruits by

auscultation. Changes can be documented by direct measurements, such as pulse volume recording.

3. Vascular calcification is often seen in X rays in late stages of atherosclerosis.

Dissection of Aorta and Rupture or Occlusion of Peripheral Arteries

These are the ultimate, tragic clinical effects of increased pressure on peripheral vessels. Diagnosis of vascular disease is apparent at that point.

The Heart

Hypertrophy

1. Left ventricular hypertrophy usually is asymptomatic.
2. Examination of the chest may reveal a forceful apical impulse palpable in the normal place over the precordium.
3. Hypertrophy can cause an extra sound (S_4), late in diastole. This is thought to be the sound made by blood hitting a thick, noncompliant ventricular wall, propelled by atrial contraction. (It is not heard in patients with atrial fibrillation.)
4. Hypertrophy is best diagnosed by echocardiography, second best by ECG. Echocardiography precisely measures ventricular wall thickness. The electrocardiogram shows increased voltage, and sometimes distortion of the ST segment and T wave when the left ventricle is hypertrophied. It is less reliable than echo.

Coronary Atherosclerosis

1. Symptoms of angina can occur, but usually not until late in the course of coronary atherosclerosis.
2. Coronary atherosclerosis is most readily detected by electrocardiography after myocardial infarction, after the disease has progressed to cause fibrosis of the ventricle, or when a "stress" is applied during the examination. ECG is not a sensitive test for coronary atherosclerosis. In fact, there are no reliable tests for atherosclerosis in its early stages.
3. Of course, it is possible to develop coronary artery disease and angina *without* hypertension, but hypertension accelerates development of angina and makes it worse. It makes angina worse by forcing the heart to work harder. "Pressure work" is more demanding on the myocardium than "output work." Hypertension requires more oxygen to generate high pressure in the left ventricle than to move blood rapidly under low pressure. Therefore, hypertension aggravates the pain of angina, just

as driving any muscle would cause pain if its circulation were impaired.

Heart Failure

1. Failure occurs in hypertension when the demands placed on the heart by arterial pressure exceed the heart's capacity to perform.
2. Heart failure is clearly symptomatic, causing fatigue, and fluid accumulation manifest by weight gain, dyspnea, and edema.
3. Failure is best diagnosed by chest X ray and physical examination. Look and listen for fluid in the lungs, a rapid pulse, an S_3 gallop, enlarged cardiac silhouette, peripheral edema, engorged veins, and hepato-jugular reflux.

The Kidneys

Nocturia and polyuria are the first symptoms of renal impairment. A failing kidney cannot concentrate urine.

Urinalysis can reveal proteinuria, and occasionally the presence of red cells, white cells or casts in cases of hypertensive renal disease.

Blood chemistry shows increased BUN and creatinine levels in severe cases of renal disease. A more sensitive test is the creatinine clearance. Clearance drops before blood chemistries rise to abnormal levels.

Late in renal disease, the kidneys are small when examined radiographically by intravenous pyelography. Early hypertensive nephropathy does not affect the appearance of the kidneys on IVP.

The Brain

Symptoms in hypertensives with brain damage are usually subtle and hard to differentiate from those of aging or psychiatric disease. There is evidence that the vascular changes of hypertension may *reduce cerebration,* as measured in intelligence and other psychological tests. Patients or their associates may note this as impaired memory.

Hypertensive patients may have *transient ischemic attacks* (TIAs), with syncope, temporary visual changes, transient paralyses or numbness, mental, or emotional changes, all of which clear completely after a few minutes or hours.

Neurologic changes detectable by physical exam occur late in the course of the disease, and result from infarcts or hemorrhage (i.e., strokes). Sometimes, the vascular event itself is unnoticed, but the residual deficit is apparent at a subsequent examination.

Symptoms of Hypertension Per Se

It is widely believed that uncomplicated, essential hypertension is "asymptomatic." Yet certain symptoms such as headache are also said to reflect the existence of an elevated pressure. Both statements are correct. A few symptoms *are* more common in hypertension, but *only slightly* more common.

Studies of symptoms in patients before and after treatment show that about one in three hypertensives have *headaches* before treatment and that half of them get better on treatment. In the control group, one in six complained of headaches. This is *not* enough of a difference to enable the examiner to conclude that the headaches are caused by hypertension. If they go away after therapy, the case for a causal relationship is stronger.

Another symptom that occurs more frequently in untreated hypertensives than in those on treatment or normals is "*blurred vision*."

A surprisingly large proportion (35%) of *untreated* hypertensives complain of *unsteadiness on standing up*. This is also a common side effect of treatment. Its occurrence in *un*treated patients may be surprising.

Overall Assessment

The World Health Organization (WHO) suggests classifying hypertensive patients into three groups. You may encounter this classification in articles about hypertension.

1. High blood pressure without evidence of organic changes in the cardiovascular system.
2. High blood pressure with cardiac hypertrophy, but without other evidence of organ damage.
3. High blood pressure with evidence of organ damage attributable to the hypertension.

Therapy Considerations

The major therapeutic considerations are (1) *whether* to treat; (2) what *modality* to use; and, if pharmacologic treatment is chosen as the modality; (3) *which drugs* to employ.

Whether to treat and whether to go to drugs involve judgments based on the *level of pressure*, the probable *susceptibility to target organ damage*, and the ability of the patient to *adhere to a diet* or other forms of therapy. (More about this in Chapter 13.)

Facts that will facilitate a decision about *whether or not to treat* are those that reflect the risk of developing atherosclerosis. Each risk factor *multiplies* the likelihood of trouble. The clinician should answer these questions:

1. Is there a family history of early vascular death or disease (such as heart attacks or strokes)?
2. Does the patient smoke?
3. Does the patient have hyperlipidemia?
4. Does the patient have hyperglycemia?
5. Is the patient obese?
6. Is the patient young and thus likely to shorten his/her life by many years because of hypertension? (See Fig. 1 in Chapter 13, for an idea of the life-shortening effects of hypertension discovered at various ages.)
7. Is the patient at high risk because of race and/or sex?

Choice of Drugs

This will depend on the likelihood of encountering *side effects* as well as on the efficacy of the drug. As will become apparent from the chapters on drugs, the clinician should inquire in advance about the presence of gout, asthma, heart block, angina, depression, etc. Each of these would rule *out* one or more commonly used drugs. General considerations such as the patient's frequency of exercise, need for alertness at work, and sexual habits and wishes will also affect the drug choice.

Summary

The workup of a patient with elevated pressure is designed to establish a *pressure* baseline, detect *curable* causes, assess past *damage,* and guide future *therapy*.

The workup can be done in either a problem-oriented way, focusing on the hypertension, or interdigitated into the traditional history-and-physical. In either case, the guidelines in this chapter should help the clinician's thinking.

13 Introduction to Therapy

Introduction

Hypertension is very dangerous to your health! In this chapter are some data to prove that point, and some guidelines to action. Figure 1 shows the effects of various pressures, occurring in men and women of different ages, on longevity. It is apparent that small increments of pressure, arising at relatively young ages, can shorten lifespan by many years.

Now the good news: Fig. 2 shows that therapy can reverse some of the life-shortening effects of hypertension. In this study, hypertensive men with diastolic pressures between 90 and 115 were either treated with drugs or not at all. The results clearly show that drug therapy reduced the incidence of such life-threatening events as stroke, heart failure, and renal disease. The results were so dramatic that the study was discontinued to spare the control group. This and other clinical trials have established beyond a doubt the positive benefits of therapy for hypertension. The only remaining questions for individual patients are (1) the level at which to initiate treatment; (2) the level of pressure to aim at during therapy; and (3) the mode of therapy.

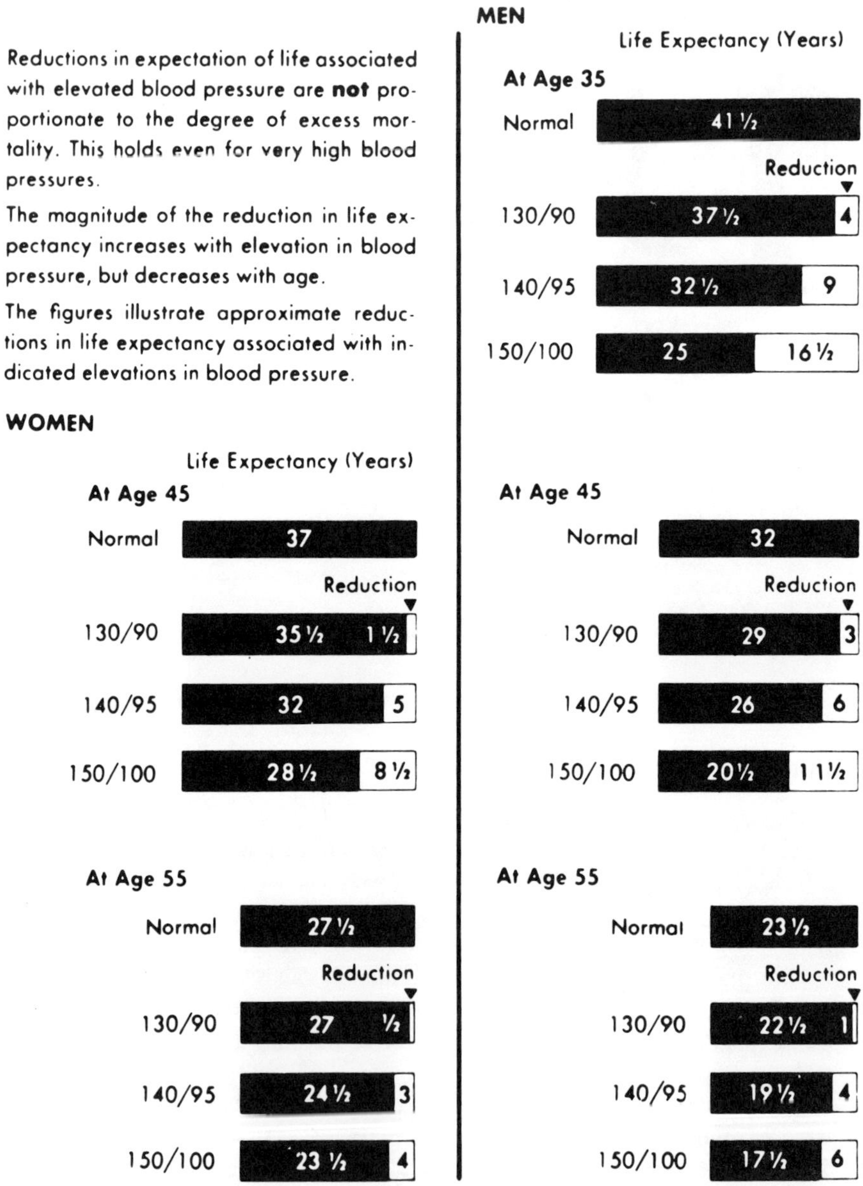

Fig. 1. Shortening of lifespan by elevated blood pressure detected at different ages in men and women. Note how drastic is the reduction in life expectancy caused by elevations of pressure that many people consider to be within the normal range. (Estimates by Statistical Bureau, Metropolitan Life Insurance Company, based on experience of 26 companies, 1935 to 1954.)

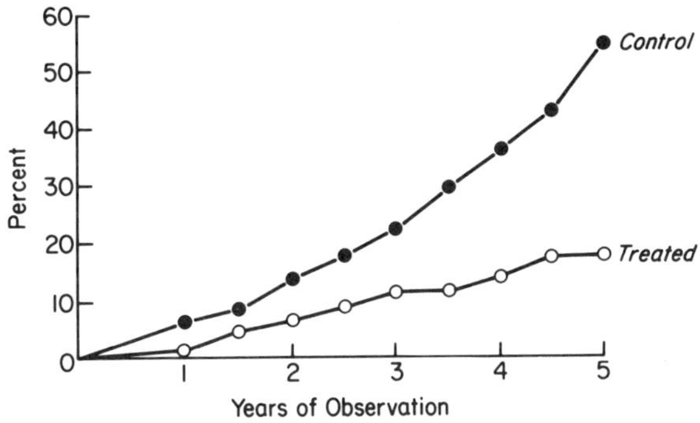

Fig. 2. Effect of drug treatment on percent of patients developing cardiovascular complications. Subjects were men with diastolic blood pressures between 90 and 114 mm Hg. Cardiovascular complications included stroke, myocardial infarction, renal failure, malignant hypertension, heart failure, etc. (from Veterans Admin. Coop. Study Group, 1970.)

When To Treat

The decision about when to treat is very complicated. In theory, *everyone* would live longer if their blood pressure were lowered; even those whose initial pressure is 120/80! The ultimate decision is based on a judgment of benefit-to-risk ratio. However, both elements in this ratio are changing constantly.

The "benefit" of treatment appears to be greater at high pretreatment pressure. However, as clinical trials use bigger and bigger groups, they can see more clearly the small decrements in morbidity and mortality that treatment can accomplish in people with relatively slight abnormalities in pressure. In addition, the "risk" of treatment diminishes as treatment becomes less toxic.

Thus, as our knowledge grows, the benefit rises, and the risk drops. This encourages more and more treatment of "borderline" cases. Still, there is understandable reluctance to use drugs to treat asymptomatic people, especially when they are elderly or very young.

It is clearly *crucial to know the pressure accurately* and to *follow it carefully!* Unless the pressure is clearly at a dangerous level, do not begin treatment until pressures have been obtained at three visits.

Monitor the patient with *home pressures* whenever possible. This not only gives you more data, and tells you what the patient is carrying in the way of pressure most of the time, but it motivates the patient and involves him/her in the treatment.

There are some patient characteristics that push you toward treatment when the pressures themselves are borderline. Treatment should be initiated for the following cases:

1. Everyone whose diastolic is 100 or greater
2. Any hypertensive (diastolic above 90 or systolic above 140) who *already has target organ damage,* for example, retinal changes, left ventricular hypertrophy, renal impairment, or neurological deficits
3. Mild hypertensives (diastolic of 90 or higher) with *two or more of the following:*
   a. Systolic pressure over 165
   b. Family history of premature cardiovascular disease
   c. The smoking habit
   d. Hyperlipidemia
   e. Hyperglycemia
   f. Age under 45
   g. Male sex
   h. Black race

The above guidelines are not absolute. The clinician can decide to start treatment in those with less disease, or omit treatment even when "indicated," based on intuition, discussions with the patient, and the ease of lowering the pressure. Although it is logical to delay treatment in patients with mild hypertension who seem to be going through a trying life situation, there are those who think of blood pressure the way we think of smoking and radiation—in terms of "pressure days" (by analogy with "pack-years" of cigarettes or rads of total body radiation). If every little bit of hypertension hurts the vessels, it would be logical to treat all cases of labile or transient hypertension. However, this seems too extreme an attitude to maintain, one that would lead to excessive drug use. If the practitioner could successfully impose nondrug interventions, such as dietary restriction of salt or relaxation techniques, he/she could treat more transient and borderline hypertension with safety. If nondrug therapy works, use it.

How Vigorously To Treat

Should every clinician aim for a target pressure of 120/80 on treatment? Again, the answer changes each year. A recent study by NIH, the Hypertension Detection and Follow-up Program (HDFP), found fewer deaths among those treated vigorously who achieved a diastolic pressure of 81 than among those treated more casually whose diastolic pressure fell to 86. These results are shown in Table I of Chapter 21. This study has changed many practitioners' attitudes, and some now advocate a target pressure of 120/80 in everyone under age 65.

In contrast to the HDFP study, the results of other experiments show little or no benefit from vigorous drug treatment of *mild* hypertension. In fact, one controversial result suggests a harmful effect of drug treatment. This is a question fraught with controversy. It is especially vexing since the number of patients with *mild* hypertension is very large compared to the number with moderate or severe elevations of pressure. It is not clear at this time that the average, uncomplicated patient would live a healthier, longer life by taking drugs to lower his/her pressure to 120/80 as compared to 130/90. In other words, the epidemiologic data showing that people with those two pressures live different life-spans can not be extrapolated to prove that drugs should be used to lower the higher pressure to the lower one. This is analogous to the finding that currently available drugs that lower blood lipids do not impose greater longevity on people with moderate elevations in serum cholesterol, even though people who naturally have low cholesterol may live longer than those with high cholesterol.

What is the safe, sensible course to take? First of all, there is no harm in establishing a *tentative* target of 120/80 for everyone (emphasis on the "tentative"). Such a target should be modified to 140 or 150/80 for people over 65, because their atherosclerotic vessels will not permit the achieving of a normal systolic pressure without lowering the diastolic to dangerous levels.

Second, institute nondrug regimens, such as weight-loss, sodium restriction, aerobic exercise, and so forth. These are very safe and often effective. (This step also permits the passage of time, which alone can solve the problem!)

Third, evaluate the patient's need for drugs based on the criteria enumerated above, with emphasis on target organ damage that may be present and patient susceptibility to atherosclerosis.

Fourth, begin drug therapy if the pressure and other factors indicate it. (Notice how vague this recommendation is!)

Finally, reassess the goal of reaching target pressure if drug side effects supervene before the goal is reached. It is better to keep patients under care at above-normal pressures than to ruin their lives or drive them away from all health care. There is some evidence that "inadequate" treatment confers significant protection from cardiovascular damage despite the persistence of above-normal pressures.

Nondrug Treatments

Diet

A diet low in *sodium* and moderate in *calories* is worth recommending to *all* hypertensives. It cannot do them any harm, and it may well do them good.

TABLE I

Salt in Foods[a]

Food	*Amount*	*Sodium (mEq)*
Bacon	1 strip	2
Baking powder	1 tsp	14
Baking soda	1 tsp	59
Beef (lean)	1 oz	1
Corned beef	1 oz	21
Beer	12 oz	1
Biscuits, baking powder	1 biscuit (2 in.)	10
Bouillon	1 cup	34
Bread (white)	1 slice	5
Canned meat	1 oz	16
Canned soup	1 cup	40–45
Canned vegetables	1 cup	10–15
Catsup	1 tbsp	7
Cheese		
natural	1 oz	9
natural, cream	1 oz	3
processed	1 oz	15–20
Chow Mein	½ cup	13
Cold cuts	1 oz	17
Cookies	1 cookie	3
Cornflakes	1 cup	7
Crackers		
"saltine"	5	7
graham	2	4
Doughnut	1	8
Dried beef	1 oz	56
Frankfurter	1	24
French fries, salted	½ cup	12
Ham (cured)	1 oz	14
Jello	½ cup	3
Milk		
whole	8 oz	5
buttermilk	8 oz	9
Pickle relish	2 tsp	6
Pie, fruit	⅛ of pie	20
Pizza	1 piece	28
Potato	1	0.1
Potato chips	1 oz	4
Pot pie (beef, etc.)	1	40–45
Pretzels, small	5	11
Rice, noodles, pasta	1 cup	0.1
Salad dressing, French	1 tbsp	9

TABLE I—*Continued*

Food	*Amount*	*Sodium (mEq)*
Salad dressing, Italian	1 tbsp	14
Salmon, regular, canned	1 oz	7
Sardines, canned	1 oz	11
Sauerkraut	½ cup	24
Sausage	1 oz	13
Soy sauce	1 tbsp	50
Sweet roll	1	9
Tomato juice, regular, canned	½ cup	10
Tomato paste	½ cup	2
Tuna, regular, canned in oil	1 oz	10
TV dinner	1	30–60
V-8 juice	½ cup	10
Vegetables, fresh (beans, corn, peas)	1 cup	0.1
Waffle, homemade	1 section (4 in.)	13
Worchestershire sauce	1 tbsp	11

[a] Note: Listings are in terms of milliequivalents (mEq) of sodium. 100 mEq = 2.3 gm sodium (5.7 gm salt).

Diet alone can successfully lower pressure in the majority of hypertensives, and in many patients, diet alone can *normalize* blood pressure.

The "no-salt added diet" (NSA) is relatively easy to achieve. It contains 4–6 gm of salt or 2 gm of sodium (100 mEq) per day and is based on the following rules:

1. Avoid "prepared" foods, i.e., those purchased in ready-to-eat form, such as "TV dinners." In general, canned foods contain more sodium (and less potassium) than frozen foods, and frozen contain more sodium than fresh foods. It is hard to believe how much salt is added during food product manufacture. Table I lists some examples.
2. Avoid excessive amounts of baked goods, milk, and milk products. Baked goods contain baking soda and baking powder; both are sodium salts. Milk contains about 20 mEq of salt per quart.
3. Never add salt (sodium chloride) during cooking or at the table. Use other spices and/or a salt substitute.

Not only does salt restriction have some value of its own, but it also potentiates all other therapy and reduces the hypokalemic side effect of diuretics (see Chapter 14).

Caloric restriction sufficient to lower weight in obese subjects is a very good treatment for hypertension! Blood pressure starts to fall when dieting begins, long before ideal weight is achieved. It seems that the "over-eating" state has a hypertensive effect all its own. (Perhaps insulin secreted in response to food intake exerts a salt-retaining effect. Obesity is always accompanied by high blood insulin, which falls quickly when food intake is reduced.)

Weight loss not only lowers blood pressure, it simultaneously removes another cardiovascular risk factor, obesity. It also makes it easier to reduce salt intake by reducing the total amount of food.

Relaxation and Exercise

Small but significant reductions in pressure can result from physical conditioning and from various relaxation techniques.

To maintain the lowered pressure, relaxation or exercise regimens must be religiously pursued. This may be harder to do than remembering to take pills. The degree of pressure reduction is slight (5–10 mm Hg), but may be adequate to return mild hypertension to normal. Remember, exercise has its own risks (e.g., trauma).

Avoid isometric exercise. It *raises* pressure acutely and dramatically in some hypertensives and can be dangerous. It is especially risky for an older hypertensive to indulge in isometric exercise.

Clenching one hand to 50% of maximum grip for only one minute can raise pressure by 50 mm Hg in a hypertensive. (It has much less effect in normals.) This is mediated by a reflex primarily involving the baroreceptors. After the muscles relax, the pressure comes down within minutes, and there is no long-term effect. (Some exercise "freaks" engaged in muscle building also take steroid hormones to accelerate development. This may also aggravate the hypertensive effect of their weight lifting.)

Isometric exercises include weight lifting, use of spring-loaded gadgets, and use of anything that tends to make you clench your teeth and hold your breath. By contrast, isotonic exercises with beneficial cardiovascular effects include such activities as swimming, cycling, and jogging (also called "aerobic" exercises). Aerobic exercises can raise systolic pressure acutely. Diastolic pressure may even fall during exercise. The long-term effect of aerobic exercise is a lowering of both systolic and diastolic pressures between exercise periods.

Follow-Up

Whether treatment involves drugs or not, the results and side effects must be monitored. The best way to monitor pressure is to instruct the patient in the use of the cuff and then have *pressures recorded at home.*

Compliance with the prescribed regimen must be assessed. Ask the patient to bring in the pill bottles. Count the pills as a rough check on how faithfully they have been taken.

Weight should be recorded at each office visit in order to note effects of diet and to detect the fluid retention that can complicate treatment.

Salt ingestion can be monitored by measuring salt excretion. The best measurement is the sodium in a 24-hr urine collection. This will be very close to the amount of sodium ingested that day. Measure creatinine in the same sample to correct for any losses.

Other Risk Factors

Hypertension is a health problem because it damages various target organs. Chief among these are the arteries. In the arteries, the major pathologic process accelerated by hypertension is atherosclerosis. (Another is rupture.) If a magic cure for atherosclerosis were invented, it would be much less urgent to treat hypertension. Although not magical, there are ways to reduce the rate of development of atherosclerosis, by controlling other *risk factors*.

Each risk factor multiplies the effects of others. (This is shown in Fig. 3.) Eliminating one risk factor reduces the damage done by the others. This is a concept that some patients would like to ignore. Some fatalists assume that one risk factor determines lifespan, and they can ignore the others. Not so. It is even *more* important to control other risk factors when one is already present. For example, the risk factor that does most damage to the heart in middle-aged men is *smoking*. Patients with or without hypertension should be urged to stop smoking. Apparently, it is the nicotine and carbon monoxide that hurts the heart and vessels, not the (cancer-causing) tars.

Do not throw up your hands and despair of ever separating a smoker from his habit. In fact, patient compliance with the instruction to "stop smoking" is about as good as compliance with the instruction to "take these pills exactly as prescribed." People tend to obey health instructions when they want to, but it takes a true act of faith to obey when it involves cessation of pleasure or commencement of expensive discomfort, all on behalf of an unseen, future gain.

A high level of blood fat is another factor that accelerates atherosclerosis. It is not proven that drugs which lower serum cholesterol and triglycerides are very effective in delaying death from atherosclerosis. They add problems from side effects as they lower plasma lipids. However, *dietary* regimens with low animal fat apparently work. They are difficult to maintain, especially in our cattle-consuming culture; but in nations forced to endure low animal fat diets (such as during war) or encouraged to do so (such as Finland in recent years), the incidence of coronary artery disease has fallen.

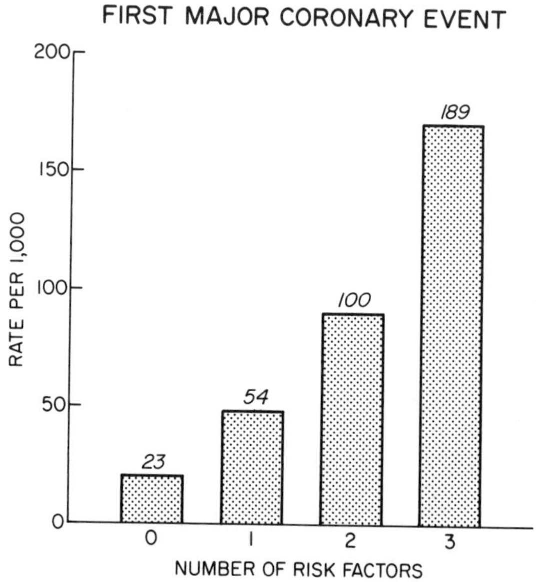

Fig. 3. Effects of hypertension, smoking, and hypercholesterolemia on myocardial infarction (from Pooling Projects, 1978). Note how each risk factor *multiplies* the damaging effects of the others. This illustrates the importance of attacking as many risk factors as possible in hypertensive patients. In this study of over 7000 middle-aged men, hypertension was defined as a diastolic pressure over 90 mm Hg, smoking was cigarette smoking of any amount, and hypercholesterolemia was a serum cholesterol level over 250 mg/dl.

Other risk factors for atherosclerosis (e.g., inheritance and gender) are a bit harder to control.

Remember, you are treating hypertension to retard atherosclerosis. Do whatever you can in addition to reducing pressure that will achieve the same goal.

Introduction to Drug Treatment

Drugs used to treat hypertension fall into three classes: diuretics, autonomic nervous system agents, and vasodilators. (The new inhibitors of angiotensin-converting enzyme are a distinct class, but they can also be thought of as vasodilators.) This division into three classes reflects our understanding of the three main organs regulating blood pressure (aside from the heart): kidneys, nervous system, and arteries themselves. The kidneys regulate body fluid volumes. The autonomic nervous system integrates the reflex control of cardiac output and vessel resistance. The resistance arteries are a target of autonomic impulses and humoral constrictors. Each one of these is blunted by one of the classes of drugs.

In Chapter 20, the "stepped-care" approach to drug treatment is described. It involves sequential addition of one drug from each class if the previous steps fail to control pressure. Thus, it is useful to divide drugs into classes not only for understanding, but in order to plan progressive steps in therapy.

Because we do not know the specific cause of hypertension in 95% of cases, we are restricted to *empiric therapies* that lower pressure. These all attack normal pressure-sustaining systems. Therefore, they all are prone to cause side effects. The miracle about antihypertensive drug therapy is that it so often normalizes pressure *without* side effects, and reduces mortality and morbidity without correcting the underlying cause of the disease.

Drug treatment can easily build on top of nondrug treatment. It is important to enlist the patient's continued cooperation in his/her care, even though the initiation of drug therapy may signal to the patient that you and your "herbs" are "taking over." Patients will require fewer drugs and suffer fewer side effects if they continue to ingest less salt and fewer calories and to indulge in moderate exercise.

All of the antihypertensive drugs available in the United States actually lower blood pressure. The FDA sees to that. Therefore, the major challenge to the clinician is to use a therapy that achieves normal pressure with the *fewest side effects*. It is helpful to know how a given drug works (or is thought to work), but from a clinical point of view, knowledge of side effects and how to minimize them is much more important.

In predicting and monitoring side effects of pressure-lowering drugs, it is helpful to think of the benefits of arterial blood pressure. These will be compromised by drugs that lower pressure, unless the drugs have a second action that compensates for the pressure drop. The beneficial effects of normal arterial pressure include the following:

1. Blood under pressure perfuses our brains, and permits changes in position or exercise. Pressure-lowering drugs often cause POSTURAL HYPOTENSION, sudden drops in pressure when patients stand up, with symptoms ranging from dizziness to syncope.
2. Blood under pressure perfuses the kidneys and enables excretion of urea, other wastes, and sodium. If pressure is inadequate, urea and other WASTES ACCUMULATE and their levels rise in the plasma. Inadequate excretion of sodium does not cause its serum concentration to rise. Instead, water is also retained, so that total FLUID VOLUME GOES UP while serum sodium concentration stays contant.
3. Blood under pressure perfuses the heart, especially in diastole. A

precipitous fall in diastolic pressure can starve the heart, especially if the coronary vessels are narrow. This can aggravate SYMPTOMS OF CORONARY ATHEROSCLEROSIS (e.g., angina).

Analysis of antihypertensive drugs must include an assessment of their effects on the brain, kidneys, and heart. At the very least, treatment of hypertension must preserve the functions of those organs.

14 Diuretics

Renal Sodium Excretion

In brief, sodium excretion is the difference between filtration of plasma through the glomerulus into the tubular urine and reabsorption of sodium from tubular urine into peritubular capillaries. All diuretics used to treat hypertension cause increased sodium excretion by inhibiting tubular reabsorption, not by increasing glomerular filtration. Different types of diuretics inhibit at different sites along the tubule. Figure 1 is an outline of diuretic action and some of its consequences.

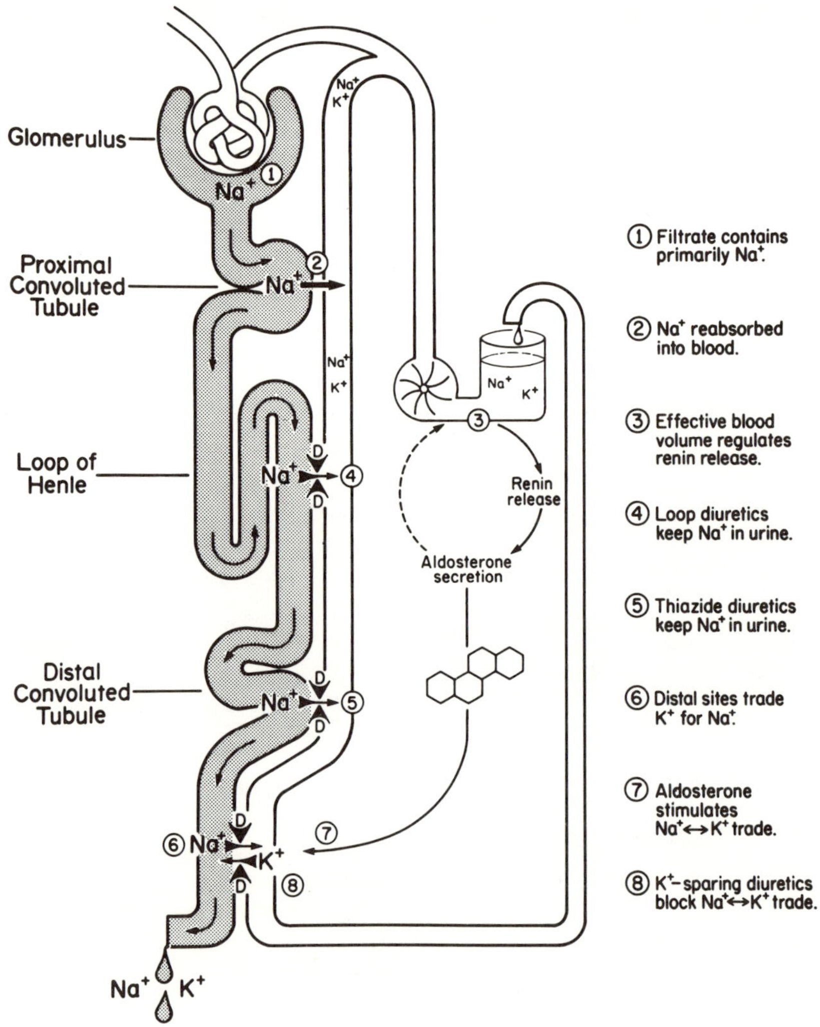

Fig. 1. Schematic representation of sodium handling by the kidneys, showing where diuretics work. By inhibiting reabsorption, thiazides and loop diuretics pass more sodium to the distal site where potassium (and H^+) are excreted in exchange for sodium. Only potassium-sparing diuretics can prevent the excessive K^+ and H^+ loss that follows diuresis. They block at the K^+-excreting distal site. Volume depletion caused by any successful diuretic accelerates K^+ and H^+ loss by stimulating the renin–angiotensin–aldosterone system.

Thiazides (e.g., Hydrochlorothiazide)

Mechanism of Hypotensive Action

By increasing excretion of sodium and water, all diuretics cause extracellular fluid *volume depletion*. This results in reduced plasma volume and reduced cardiac output. At least some of the antihypertensive effect of diuretics is the result of this volume depletion.

Volume depletion triggers renin release and activates the renin–aldosterone axis. The actions of angiotensin on blood vessels and of aldosterone on the kidney blunt and partially correct the initial volume depletion. After a few months of diuretic therapy, plasma volume is rebuilt to not-quite-normal. Despite this, pressure remains low.

Thiazides inhibit sodium reabsorption at the distal tubule (''diluting segment''). Thiazide diuretics also cause reduction in peripheral resistance. The mechanism is unknown. It may involve the actions of prostaglandins released by the diuretic. Another possible mechanism is a reduction in reactivity of vessels to pressor agents. Sodium depletion, by any means, causes reduced vascular reactivity.

Side Effects

1. Hypokalemia (Serum K^+ Concentration <3.5 mEq/L)

By acting at the cortical diluting segment of the distal tubule, thiazides pass more sodium down to the site where aldosterone works. Thus, aldosterone release is stimulated by volume depletion, and the aldosterone-stimulated tubule sees a great deal of sodium it can reabsorb in exchange for potassium. This leads to the potassium loss that characterizes thiazide diuretic use (see Fig. 1).

Hypokalemia occurs to some degree in about half the people taking thiazides. It is more likely to occur at higher doses and in people who have preexisting elevated adrenal steroid secretion (e.g., people with aldosteronoma's).

Severe hypokalemia can cause weakness of muscles, muscle cramps, and reduced capacity of the kidneys to concentrate urine (which in turn causes nocturia). The levels of potassium at which these side effects occur vary widely. It is uncommon to see them at serum levels above 3.5 mEq/L.

The hypokalemia of diuretic use may be accompanied by a mild alkalosis, like that of primary aldosteronism (''hypokalemic alkalosis''). This is caused by excretion of H^+ as well as K^+ at the site where aldosterone works.

Hypokalemia has always been considered particularly dangerous when digitalis is administered, because the arrhythmias that complicate digitalis are much more likely to occur when the serum K^+ is low. There is recent evidence that arrhythmias are more common in people who suffer a myocardial infarction while their serum K^+ is below 4.0, *whether digitalis is being given or not*. In fact, there is even evidence that ventricular premature beats are unusually frequent in typical, healthy hypertensives with thiazide-induced hypokalemia. The significance of all this ventricular "ectopy" is hard to gauge, but it cannot be doing any good! It suggests that one should always avoid, or treat, thiazide-induced hypokalemia. A more conservative approach is to treat hypokalemia in the following cases: (1) patients taking digitalis, (2) patients with symptoms likely to be caused by low K^+ levels, (3) patients with frequent extra systoles, and (4) patients with serum K^+ levels below 3.0 mEq/L. Treatment of hypokalemia is described in the next chapter, but we may begin by mentioning that therapy can include potassium supplements, potassium-sparing diuretics, or captopril to block the renin–angiotensin–aldosterone system.

2. Hyperuricemia

Hyperuricemia occurs in over half the people taking thiazides. Virtually everyone's uric acid rises somewhat, but not to abnormal levels. If uric acid levels *do not* go up 1 mg/dl, the patient is probably not taking the thiazide!

Hyperuricemia is not a problem unless gouty attacks occur. (Although theoretically possible, damage to the kidneys probably does not occur with diuretic-induced hyperuricemia.)

Treat diuretic-induced hyperuricemia with probenecid or allopurinol or by switching from thiazide to another class of hypotensive drug, but do this only when gouty attacks occur or when uric acid levels rise above 12 mg/dl.

3. Hyperglycemia

Decreased glucose tolerance is a minor side effect of thiazide use, but it is noticed frequently because of the wide use of SMA-12 and other automated blood analyzers. Diabetics may require a higher dose of hypoglycemic medication when taking thiazides. Latent diabetics may "come out of the closet" when on thiazides.

4. Hyperlipidemia

About 50% of patients on thiazide diuretics have a significant rise in serum LDL cholesterol and triglyceride levels. The mechanism is unknown, but may involve inhibition of insulin secretion. It is most dramatic in diabetics. This could be a very important side effect. It would partially negate the benefit of antihypertensive treatment in reducing cardiovascular morbidity.

5. Hypercalcemia

Thiazides *reduce renal excretion* of Ca^{2+}. This can be useful in treating urinary stones, but the reduced excretion may *raise the blood* calcium level.

Note: Loop diuretics (described below) do exactly the *opposite,* i.e., causing calcium diuresis. Therefore, one should use thiazides to treat *urinary* calcium stones and loop diuretics to treat high *blood* calcium.

6. Postural Hypotension and/or Extreme Sodium Depletion

These can occur when thiazides (or any other diuretic) are used. These problems are most bothersome in the elderly; postural hypotension probably occurs much more often than we think, and clearly limits the use of diuretic therapy in the aged. Extreme sodium depletion, with low serum sodium, causes weakness and unusual mental changes. It is easy to correct, but hard to recognize on purely clinical grounds.

7. Other Side Effects

Pancreatitis. Thiazides are one of the drugs to suspect as a cause of pancreatitis. The mechanism is unknown. Do not prescribe thiazides for patients with a history of pancreatitis.

Sensitivity to sunlight. Some patients tan in the sun more readily when taking thiazides.

Reduced renal function. Renal failure can be aggravated by thiazides. In cases of impaired renal function, when the serum creatinine is greater than 2.0 mg/dl, use loop diuretics. (They increase renal blood flow).

Reduced hepatic function. This condition can be aggravated by thiazides or any diuretic. In its extreme form, this side effect can lead to hepatic coma. The mechanism is probably related to reduced circulation to the liver. Diuretics are a notorious cause of "hepatorenal syndrome," simultaneous failure of kidneys and liver, in patients with very badly diseased livers. This is not a problem in otherwise healthy patients.

Diarrhea. Diarrhea can result from diuretic use. In cases of intractable diarrhea, consider the possibility that the patient is sensitive to diuretics or is taking them in excessive amounts to reduce weight or feign illness.

Use in Treatment of Hypertension

Thiazide diuretics are still the best drugs to use to begin treatment of hypertension of all kinds. They are the foundation of therapy—cheap, effective, and well understood. Thiazides may be adequate by themselves to treat about half of all *mild* hypertensives.

The combination of low-salt diet *and* diuretics is more hypotensive than either alone. Furthermore, low salt intake lessens the likelihood of hypokalemia. (However, adequate diuretic dosage may enable a hypertensive to eat some salt and get away with it!)

The full effect of thiazides on blood pressure may not be seen for 2 weeks or longer. Try not to change the dose or add other drugs until each stage of therapy has been tested at least 2 weeks.

Thiazides truly potentiate all other antihypertensives. Intravascular volume depletion makes patients more susceptible to vasodilators and autonomic inhibitors that reduce cardiac output. (Furthermore, during diuretic use sensitivity to all vasoconstrictors is reduced.) When other drugs are added, thiazides should not be stopped, but the dose of diuretic may be lowered to reduce side effects.

Thiazides have a flat dose–response curve. Many people do well on one tablet per day. There is usually no increase in hypotensive effect with more than two tablets per day. A typical dose of thiazide is hydrochlorothiazide, 50 mg every morning. Although many people get a better pressure response to 50 mg b.i.d., this dose carries a higher incidence of side effects, notably hypokalemia. There are a large number of other thiazides available, but they do not improve upon hydrochlorthiazide in their ability to lower pressure.

Other Thiazide-Like Diuretics

Chlorthalidone (Hygroton®) is chemically distinct from the thiazides, but exerts very similar effects. It has a relatively long duration of action (48 hr). This makes every-other-day therapy possible, but that is a hard regimen for some patients to remember. The long duration is also potentially dangerous if daily, high doses are given and blood levels escalate. The major deleterious effect of a high blood level is hypokalemia.

The current recommendation is to use chlorthalidone at a dose of 25 mg per day or per 2 days. At that level, good pressure reduction is obtained with little hypokalemia. At higher doses, very little additional pressure reduction is obtained, but more side effects are induced.

Metolazone (Zaroxolyn® or Diulo®) is intermediate in duration between thiazides and chlorthalidone. This permits once a day dosage without cumulative effects. Aside from that, metolazone has no advantage over hydrochlorthiazide (and many patients do well on once-a-day hydrochlorothiazide).

"Loop" Diuretics: Furosemide (Lasix) and Ethacrynic Acid (Edecrin)

Mechanism of Action

These drugs are the most potent diuretics known. They work in the Loop of Henle to inhibit sodium and chloride reabsorption.

Loop diuretics limit the ability of the kidney to concentrate urine (because concentration requires high salt content in the interstitial space *around* the Loops of Henle). Thus, the loop diuretics cause a dramatic excretion of sodium *and* water.

Loop diuretics lower pressure at first by their effect on blood volume. After a time, these drugs also cause reduced peripheral resistance, but unlike thiazides they almost never lose their ability to shrink volume.

Side Effects

1. Like the thiazides, loop diuretics cause low serum K^+, high serum uric acid, higher blood glucose, and higher serum cholesterol levels.
2. Loop diuretics cause Ca^{2+} *diuresis*. Therefore, they are useful in treating hypercalcemia, but *bad* for urinary *stones*.
3. Loop diuretics can cause reversible *deafness* when given in high doses, especially in people with impaired renal function who may achieve very high blood levels of drug. Apparently, the loop diuretics can upset the delicate fluid balance in the cochlea.
4. Because they are so potent, loop diuretics can cause extreme *volume depletion,* resulting in postural hypotension. They also cause a great deal of prompt urine formation, which can be annoying at night or embarrassing by day.

Use in Hypertension

Furosemide and ethacrynic acid are shorter acting than thiazides. They are more potent as diuretics, but for a given diuretic effect, they are less efficacious as pressure-lowering drugs.

They are especially useful in treating hypertension in patients with renal disease or in emergencies when fast results are needed. One rule of thumb is to give loop diuretics instead of thiazides when the serum creatinine is over 2 mg/dl.

Because they have a short duration of action, loop diuretics used twice a day or less may cause *less* K^+ wastage than thiazides. Perhaps between doses the body regains K^+. (By contrast to the short duration of diuretic effect, the hypotensive effect of loop diuretics lasts up to 12 hr.) However, with more frequent administration, loop diuretics can cause even more K^+ wastage than thiazides because they are so powerful.

A typical dose of a typical loop diuretic is furosemide 20 mg every morning and at supper.

In patients with severe fluid retention that resists even the loop diuretics, a combination of loop plus thiazide or loop plus metolazone can be an effective "superdiuretic." Another trick is to add captopril which can dilate renal vessels.

Potassium-Sparing Diuretics: Spironolactone (Aldactone), Triamterene (Dyrenium), and Amiloride (Midamor)

Thiazides and loop diuretics cause K^+ wastage. In response to their effects on volume, aldosterone levels increase and K^+ is lost by the kidney trying to save Na^+. By contrast, "potassium-sparing" diuretics act further down the tubule and "spare" potassium. That is, they do not "waste" K^+ while diuresing Na^+. In addition, they can act as antidotes to the potassium wasting caused by thiazide and loop diuretics; that is their main use today.

Spironolactone

Mechanism of Action

This agent is a specific, competitive inhibitor of aldosterone. It is only effective when adrenal function is intact. It takes 1000 molecules of spironolactone to antagonize one molecule of aldosterone.

Spironolactone has some intrinsic hypotensive action, because its mild diuretic effect causes a reduction in blood volume followed by slight vasodilatation. But this action is weak, and spironolactone is seldom used alone.

The diuretic effects of spironolactone are partially blocked by aspirin. (This suggests that part of its effect is mediated by prostaglandins.)

Side Effects

1. The most worrisome side effect of spironolactone is *high* serum potassium levels (*hyper*kalemia). Hyperkalemia can be *fatal;* it can cause cardiac arrest. It is especially likely to occur in patients with renal disease or diabetes. *Do not give K^+ supplements* or "salt substitutes" when you give spironolactone or triamterene, unless you watch the serum K^+ carefully. Drugs like captopril, which lower aldosterone levels by interfering with the renin cascade, will potentiate effects of spironolactone and predispose to hyperkalemia.

2. Spironolactone can also cause gynecomastia in males, menstrual irregularities in females, and nausea in all sexes.

Use in Hypertension

The most common dose of spironolactone is 25 mg combined with 25 mg of hydrochlorothiazide (Aldactazide®) taken once or twice a day.

Triamterene

Mechanism of Action

This drug is not a competitive antagonist of aldosterone, so it works whether or not aldosterone is present. It inhibits the Na^+/K^+ exchange mechanism directly.

Side Effects

Beware high K^+ levels. Do not give K^+ along with triamterene unless the potassium level is monitored. Do not give triamterene to patients with diabetes or renal failure, for fear of hyperkalemia. Hyperkalemia is more likely to occur when triamterene and potassium supplements are given along with a converting enzyme inhibitor (such as captopril) which reduces the secretion of aldosterone.

Use in Hypertension

A common regimen contains 50 mg of triamterene in combination with 25 mg of hydrochlorothiazide (Dyazide®) in one tablet, used once or twice a day. Triamterene is such a mild diuretic it has no proven antihypertensive effect when used alone.

Amiloride

Amilonide, a new, K^+-sparing diuretic, works directly on the Na^+/K^+-ATPase of the kidney, whether or not aldosterone is present. It is a more long-lived diuretic than spironolactone or triamterene. And it is most commonly used at a dose of 5 mg in combination with 50 mg of hydrochlorothiazide (Moduretic®) given once a day.

Other Aspects

Neither spironolactone, triamterene, nor amiloride causes high uric acid or inceased blood glucose.

All three potassium-sparing agents find their major use in combination with thiazides.

Used as a second drug, a K^+-sparing diuretic has two effects: (1) it lowers pressure further because of its additive diuresis and (2) it helps maintain serum K^+ at a normal level.

Common Effects of All Diuretics

All diuretics cause initial *volume depletion*. This depletion is the effect that potentiates all other antihypertensive agents. On the other hand, volume depletion can be symptomatic, causing dizziness, weakness or blackout upon arising from a lying or sitting position. This is most serious in elderly people. Volume depletion is also dangerous in patients with advanced liver disease, and can drive them into hepatic failure.

All diuretics stimulate release of renin by the kidneys, *raise the plasma renin activity* (PRA), and invoke the compensatory mechanism initiated by renin that blunts their effectiveness.

In high doses, or after prolonged therapy, diuretics can lead to *sodium depletion*. In its full-blown form, sodium depletion can lead to low serum sodium concentrations. This condition presents clinically as weakness and abnormal mental function. People get quite "squirrely" with a low serum sodium level. It is a difficult syndrome to detect clinically, but easy to treat by reducing the diuretic dose and restricting water intake.

Drug Interactions Affecting Diuretics

Lithium is commonly used to treat manic–depressive psychosis and some other psychiatric disorders. Diuretics, especially thiazides, reduce excretion of lithium and *raise lithium levels* in the blood. So, one should reduce lithium doses by about one-third when adding a diuretic, and monitor the blood level carefully for a month or two, making fine adjustments as needed.

Nonsteroidal antiinflammatory drugs (NSAIDs) [e.g., aspirin, ibuprofen (Motrin), and indomethacin (Indocin)] reduce the antihypertensive effectiveness of diuretics. Patients whose pressures had been normalized may find their readings going up if they start to take NSAIDs. The best approach, if both are needed, is to increase the diuretic dose.

New Diuretics under Development

Several new loop diuretics are under development. They will be touted as more powerful or longer lived than furosemide, but these features may make them less useful in treating hypertension. A weaker drug with less K^+ loss might be more valuable for the hypertensive.

One new diuretic, indapamide (Lozol®), combines the antihypertensive efficacy of hydrochlorothiazide with the potency of loop diuretics. This could prove very useful in some cases.

Uricosuric diuretics that will lower rather than raise uric acid are known. Although useful in rare gouty patients, they offer no big advantage for the average hypertensive. On the other hand, a diuretic that lowered LDL cholesterol would be terrific!

15 Potassium and Magnesium

Hypokalemia (Low K^+ Levels)

Introduction

Most body potassium is in muscle and bone. Only 0.4% of the total is in serum, so the level in serum may not be a perfect reflection of the total body potassium stores. One implication of this is the need for large amounts of potassium to replete a patient whose serum potassium is only mildly depressed. Normal serum K^+ levels range from 3.5–5.0 mEq/L. A summary of factors affecting serum K^+ levels is found in Table I.

Causes

Most cases of hypokalemia result from treatment with thiazide or loop diuretics. This condition can also occur when large amounts of potassium are lost through emesis, diarrhea, or laxative over-indulgence.

Hyperaldosteronism is a rare but well-understood cause of potassium loss. In fact, it is the secondary hyperaldosteronism following volume depletion that accounts for much of the potassium loss with diuretic usage. Diuretics trigger renin release, which stimulates aldosterone secretion. The aldosterone

TABLE I

Regulation of Serum Potassium

Factors lowering K^+ *levels*	*Factors* raising K^+ *levels*
1. Increased renal excretion	1. Decreased renal excretion
A. Hyperaldosteronism	A. Adrenal insufficiency or reduced aldosterone secretion (may be induced by diabetes and worsened by drugs such as ACE inhibitors or nonsteroidal antiinflammatory drugs).
B. Thiazide or loop diuretics (plus the hyperaldosteronism they cause)	B. Renal failure
C. Antibiotics, such as carbenicillin, ticarcillin, and amphotericin	C. Potassium-sparing diuretics
2. Shift of K^+ from plasma to cells	2. Shift of K^+ from cells to plasma
A. Insulin plus glucose	A. Insulin insufficiency
B. Alkalosis (H^+ enters plasma from cells, K^+ enters cells to take its place)	B. Acidosis (H^+ goes into cells, K^+ comes out into plasma)
C. Epinephrine-induced K^+ shift into muscle	C. Possible effect of β blockers
3. Losses from bowel	3. Dietary intake
A. Diarrhea	A. Foods rich in K^+
B. Laxative excess	B. Potassium supplements
C. Vomiting	

finds a fertile field at the distal tubule. There, the diuretic has provided a great deal of sodium that can be exchanged for potassium under the influence of aldosterone. This sequence is presented schematically in Fig. 1 of Chapter 14.

Hyperaldosteronism that exists before diuretics are added, such as primary aldosteronism from an adrenal adenoma, predisposes the patient to hypokalemia that can be exaggerated by diuretics. Some clinicians use the occurrence of severe hypokalemia after thiazide administration as a clue to the existence of primary hyperaldosteronism.

Hypokalemia is made more common by the eating of processed foods, especially canned goods. Canning and other processing leaches out potassium, while at the same time the processor usually adds sodium. For example, whole flour contains three times as much potassium as processed bake goods; fresh peas contain three times as much potassium as canned peas (and 0.5% as much sodium!); and fresh beef contains twice as much potassium as corned beef.

Consequences and Implications

Symptoms of hypokalemia include muscle weakness, muscle cramps, and nocturia. The nocturia results from a renal tubular change, "hypokalemia nephropathy." When potassium concentration is low, the tubule cannot concentrate urine as well, large volumes of dilute urine are produced, and some of this is excreted at night.

Hypokalemia secondary to diuretics is usually accompanied by a mild *alkalosis*. Hydrogen ions, as well as potassium ions, are excreted at the distal tubule. This further aggravates depletion of serum K^+ by driving K^+ into cells in place of H^+. Correction of hypokalemia is accelerated by correction of alkalosis.

The most dangerous effect of hypokalemia is cardiac *arrhythmia*. This is more likely if the patient is taking digitalis. Recently, evidence has accumulated showing higher incidence of ventricular arrhythmias, ranging from premature beats to fibrillation, in patients with lower serum potassium whether or not they take digitalis. The incidence of the arrhythmias was greater the lower the potassium level. Some of these observations were made in postmyocardial infarction patients and some in ambulatory essential hypertensives.

If confirmed, the significance of these findings to the hypertensive with known myocardial disease or digitalis therapy would be evident: one would be compelled to keep the serum level and total body potassium stores normal. The significance for young hypertensives without symptoms, those without cardiac hypertrophy, or those with marginally subnormal potassium levels is less evident. It would seem logical to err on the side of normal potassium until larger studies are completed.

Hypokalemia is a serious problem for patients undergoing general anesthesia. The low K^+ level predisposes to intraoperative arrhythmia and also potentiates the effects of muscle relaxants such as succinyl choline. As will be pointed out below, it is not adequate preoperative preparation to give potassium to a depleted patient on the night before surgery just to achieve normal morning serum K^+. Unless repletion of total body stores is achieved, the added K^+ drifts into other body fluid compartments, and the serum and muscles may again display K^+ deficiency during the day of surgery.

Prevention and Treatment

Prevention and treatment of diuretic-induced hypokalemia are achieved most dependably by the use of a diuretic mixture including a potassium-sparing diuretic (combination tablets such as Dyazide, Aldactazide, or Moduretic). Unfortunately, the combinations cost more than a thiazide alone and introduce the possible side effect of the potassium-sparing diuretics.

A new approach to hypokalemia is the use of captopril to interrupt the renin–angiotensin–aldosterone system by inhibiting angiotensin converting enzyme (ACE). This drug lowers plasma levels of aldosterone. Its use helps prevent or reverse hypokalemia aggravated by diuretics.

Prevention of hypokalemia can often be achieved by ingestion of oral potassium supplements, in the form of K^+-rich foods, tablets, or powders. Foods rich in potassium include: fruits and fruit juices (most popular are orange juice and bananas); fresh vegetables such as spinach and potatoes; nuts and seeds (NOT the salted ones, please); and fresh fish and beef.

The recommended foods may be "relatively" rich in potassium, but that is not saying much. A quart of orange juice contains only 50 mEq of K^+, a banana contains only 10. It might be possible to prevent or delay hypokalemia with food, but it is difficult to treat real K^+ depletion that way. The same complaint can be registered for potassium pills—most contain less than 10 mEq of potassium per tablet.

The richest potassium supplements are either powders that dissolve in water or ready-made solutions. Although they supply 15 to 25 mEq per dose, they do have a very bitter flavor.

Perhaps the easiest way to prevent hypokalemia is to use potassium chloride in place of sodium as a condiment. These preparations (such as Morton's Salt-Substitute and Co-Salt®) achieve two goals at once: lessening of sodium intake and replacement of potassium. Unfortunately, they taste relatively bitter, so patients often drift back to table salt. (Using salt substitutes that contain half sodium chloride and half potassium chloride is like using low-nicotine cigarettes; people tend to suck harder or ingest more to get the same net quantity of the "forbidden fruit.")

To correct the alkalosis that usually accompanies hypokalemia in patients taking thiazide or loop diuretics, it is best to replenish potassium as the chloride salt. Therefore, KCl is a better replacement salt that the better tasting gluconate or citrate salts. Correction of alkalosis with chloride can bring the serum K^+ level to normal before total body K^+ stores are replenished.

The most important lesson about potassium repletion is to use enough. One convenient rule of thumb is to assume that the patient requires at least 200 mEq total replacement for each mEq depression in serum K^+ level. That may be too little, but rarely too much. Furthermore, remember that the patient may continue to lose K^+ while you are pouring it in. The diuretic effect may last, the diarrhea may persist, and there is a predictable loss in urine and stool regardless of what else you do.

If hypokalemia is severe or difficult to correct, suspect *low magnesium* (see following).

Hyperkalemia (High K^+ Levels)

It is imperative to remember the warnings about *hyper*kalemia. Do not give potassium-sparing diuretics to patients with renal impairment and/or diabetes, unless you are doing it as a temporary measure to replete K^+. Do not give both the potassium-sparing diuretic and potassium supplements to patients with adrenal failure, renal failure, and/or diabetes. The danger of hyperkalemia is accentuated by use of converting enzyme inhibitors like captopril, which reduce aldosterone output by removing the angiotensin stimulus. A rare cause of high serum K^+ level is use of nonsteroidal antiinflammatory drugs, which can inhibit renin release, reducing aldosterone levels. In all of these instances, one runs the danger of *hyper*kalemia, a situation in which patients can experience *cardiac arrest* (an asymptomatic, but undesirable side effect!)

Hypomagnesemia

Diuretics, aldosterone excess, diarrhea, vomiting, and alcoholism can deplete the body of magnesium as well as potassium.

Like potassium, magnesium resides in cells, bone, and other body stores, with very little (0.4%) in the plasma.

Normal serum levels of magnesium are 1.5–2.5 mEq/L.

Hypomagnesemia has its own cluster of symptoms, resembling low serum calcium in many ways, including tremors, convulsions, ataxia, and cardiac arrhythmias.

Magnesium deficiency makes it very difficult to replenish potassium. Apparently, magnesium is a cofactor for the cellular apparatus that pumps K^+. Therefore, it is prudent to suspect hypomagnesemia in patients found to have low serum K^+ levels, especially those whose K^+ is hard to raise.

To replace depleted magnesium, give magnesium sulfate, a total of 12 gm by mouth over several days, or 4 gm im over one or two days. Go much slower in patients with renal failure and check the magnesium again a day or two after the last dose, when there has been time for equilibration of the body pools.

16 Drugs Acting on the Autonomic Nervous System: α Blockers and α Agonists

Introduction

It has been known for centuries that fear and excitement temporarily raise blood pressure, so it was reasonable to assume that chronic elevations of pressure were caused by chronic states of excitement, stress, or fear. When physiologists identified the autonomic nervous system as the translator of central nervous perceptions into cardiovascular responses, ways to interrupt autonomic pathways were sought as a treatment for high blood pressure. Surgical sympathectomy, performed in the 1930s and 1940s, successfully lowered blood pressure. However, the surgery also blocked autonomic reflexes, such as those originating in the baroreceptors. Patients' pressures became very labile after this surgery. Some could no longer stand or exercise without blacking out.

Recent pharmacologic approaches to the autonomic nervous system have been more successful than surgery in combining autonomic blockade with preservation of normal function. We do not yet know if this is a result of good logic or good luck. All of the assumptions on which this therapy is based are flawed, but the drugs work very well!

Conceptual Formulation of the Autonomic Nervous System

It is very useful to remember the traditional division of all nervous system phenomena into cholinergic, α adrenergic, and β adrenergic. Another traditional division is between central and peripheral autonomic events. Thus, there are central α-adrenergic phenomena, peripheral α-adrenergic phenomena, etc. The central functions are less well defined than the peripheral, and some central functions appear to be paradoxical in the light of our knowledge of peripheral events. For example, central α-adrenergic receptors mediate vasodilation; the opposite of peripheral α receptors which mediate vasoconstriction. These concepts are shown schematically in Fig. 1 of Chapter 3.

The sequence of cellular events in all nervous system functions is (1) synthesis of transmitter, (2) release of transmitter, (3) interaction of receptors with transmitter, (4) events mediated by receptor–transmitter interaction, and (5) recapture and degradation of transmitter. These events pertain to *all* divisions of the nervous system and form the basis on which drugs are designed. (Some block receptors, some block recapture of transmitter, etc.)

Ganglion-Blocking Agents

Ganglion blockers, the first drugs used specifically for treating hypertension, blocked the autonomic nervous system at the level of the sympathetic ganglia. This effectively blocked α- and β-adrenergic impulses, leaving the parasympathetic (vagal) system unopposed. A typical drug was pentolinium. By interrupting all sympathetic reflexes, they caused dramatic postural hypotension. Problems with other autonomic functions, such as diarrhea, dry mouth, and altered male sexual function, resulted from unopposed cholinergic dominance.

Ganglion blockers do *not* cross the blood–brain barrier; therefore, they cause no sedation or depression. This in itself was an appealing quality of the drugs, but not enough to keep them from falling out of favor when milder, more selective adrenergic modifiers came into use.

The only ganglion-blocking drug now used is *Arfonad*® (trimethaphan camsylate). It is used in hypertensive emergencies and in the operating room, where posture can be controlled and where autonomic side effects are manageable.

The problem with ganglion blockers is their shotgun-like effect on all autonomic functions. They do *too* much.

α-Adrenergic Blockers [e.g., Prazosin (Minipress)]

Of all the antihypertensive drugs affecting autonomic function, α blockers are the easiest to understand. Our best guess is that they selectively block the peripheral, postsynaptic, pressor effects of norepinephrine, notably vasoconstriction. (I hope that is all we ever learn about them, because at this stage of understanding they are ideal drugs to begin a discussion of autonomic modulators.)

Mechanism of Action

Prazosin and drugs like it are blockers of α_1 receptors, the classical postsynaptic receptors on the far side of the cleft that stimulate vascular smooth muscle contraction.

Prazosin has a relatively large effect on the *visceral* arterial bed, causing some pooling of blood there.

Prazosin also has some effect on the CNS, but most of its antihypertensive effect appears to be peripheral.

Prazosin is a pure α_1 antagonist. It does *NOT* block α_2 (presynaptic) receptors. As a result, released norepinephrine swings back in the synapse, binds to its own presynaptic sites, and turns off its own synthesis. With less norepinephrine synthesis, there is less free norepinephrine released into the circulation where it could reach the heart. Thus, there is less compensatory tachycardia.

Prazosin decreases release of renin by the kidneys. (Note: Both β blockers and α blockers reduce renin release.)

Side Effects

1. *Postural hypotension* can be dramatic with the *first dose* of prazosin in about 5% of patients. After the first dose, postural hypotension is a less dramatic problem, but it can still be bothersome.
2. *CNS symptoms* include drowsiness, headache, and vertigo.
3. *Fluid retention* (unless diuretics are given) is the result of reduced pressure in the renal circulation, as Guyton's formulation would have

predicted. Although renal vessels may dilate, the head of arterial pressure may fall enough to reducc glomerular filtration pressure.

Use in Hypertension

Prazosin is effective in most hypertensives, but the magnitude of its effect is frequently small, about equal to that of thiazides. To get a bigger effect, the dose must be advanced to the point where postural hypotension can become limiting. Like all other drugs affecting blood vessels, Prazosin's effects are potentiated by administration of diuretics. It is rarely used alone.

Prazosin is logical to add to a regimen of diuretic plus a β blocker such as propranolol in patients with peripheral vascular insufficiency. These patients can get into trouble from excess α-adrenergic vasoconstriction in their limbs when β blockers leave α-adrenergic influences unopposed.

Prazosin is ideal treatment for patients with pheochromocytoma before surgery or when surgery is impossible. It is important to block α receptors before tampering with the tumor.

Prazosin has been reported to reduce the bronchoconstriction some asthmatics experience on strenuous exercise. (This could be helpful in cases where β blockers tend to aggravate bronchoconstriction.)

One should always *START PRAZOSIN SLOWLY*. Use 1.0 mg as the initial dose and watch for postural pressure drop. Prescribe the first dose to be given at night after the patient is *actually in bed!* This First Dose Effect is unexplained. Once over that obstacle, patients become less susceptible to the drug, and need their dose titrated up. The First Dose Effect has scared some physicians into using no greater than a tiny dose of prazosin in all hypertensives. Actually, some people require hefty doses to obtain beneficial results.

One should titrate prazosin dose up from 1.0 mg to as much as 10.0 mg per dose, orally, two to three times daily. Use it in combination with a diuretic, or with a diuretic plus a β blocker.

Other α Blockers

Phenoxybenzamine, one of the oldest α blockers, is potent, but causes a great deal of postural hypotension and tachycardia. (This drug blocks both α_1 and α_2 receptors, so norepinephrine synthesis is increased.) Phenoxybenzamine is effective by the oral route.

Phentolamine (Regitine) is a short-acting α blocker given intravenously. Its most common use has been to help in the diagnosis of pheochromocytoma. It is also a handy intravenous emergency medication for treating pheochromocytoma, clonidine withdrawal (see below), or norepinephrine overdose.

Labetalol is a combined α and β blocker. It is new to the United States, but has been used widely overseas. Postural hypotension limits its usefulness in some patients.

Trimazosin is a prazosin analog currently being tested. It is longer acting than prazosin, but still has a First Dose Effect in some patients.

Other Uses of α Blockers

Prazosin, its analogs, and other drugs that dilate arteries can be used to relieve the heart of its need to pump against high resistance. Such "afterload" reduction can help failing hearts and actually increase cardiac output and the perfusion of other organs. We will discuss it again under Hypertensive Crises (Chapter 22).

α-Adrenergic Agonists

Methyldopa [α-Methyldopa (Aldomet)]

Mechanism of Action

Originally designed to block dopa decarboxylase, methyldopa now appears to exert its antihypertensive action in the CNS, after transformation to α-methyldopamine and α-methylnorepinephrine. α-Methyldopamine and α-methylnorepinephrine are weak analogs of dopamine and norepinephrine and have been called "false neurotransmitters."

α-Methylnorepinephrine, by contrast with norepinephrine, is relatively specific for turning on α_2 receptors, the presynaptic receptors that *turn off* norepinephrine synthesis, and the receptors in CNS centers that reduce pressor impulses. So the metabolite of methyldopa selectively hits the pressure-lowering receptors.

The hypotensive effects of methyldopa can be blocked experimentally by administration of α-receptor *blockers* into the CNS. Thus, the pressure-lowering effect of the drug depends on its ability to *turn on α receptors in the brain*. As a result of altered nerve traffic from the brain, *peripheral resistance falls* with methyldopa.

There is maintenance of renal blood flow during methyldopa therapy, despite the fall in blood pressure, indicating some vasodilation of the renal vascular bed. However, the vasodilation in the renal vessels is not enough to compensate fully for the fall in pressure, so some fluid retention is seen. In other words, it appears that glomerular filtration pressure falls despite some dilatation of renal vessels.

Renin release is reduced by methyldopa. This may contribute to its pressure-lowering effect.

There is relatively *little* postural hypotension with methyldopa and no change in cardiac output or pulse after the drug is given. In general, drugs acting on the *CNS* work *smoothly* to lower pressure and *maintain cardiovascular reflexes* for moment-to-moment pressure control.

Side Effects

1. Sedation. A common problem with all CNS-active drugs, this side effect can "creep up" on people and affect them without their connecting it to the drug. People seem to get used to the feeling, or suffer less sedation as time passes, despite continuation of the drug.
2. Impotence. This side effect is common in drug treatment of hypertension and has caused more noncompliance than you can shake a stick at! It is hard to tell how much impotence is the result of a patient's concern over being sick, sedation by drugs, lower pressure *per se,* or a specific side effect of a given drug. Clearly, those drugs affecting the brain, like methyldopa, cause some cases of impotence. The problem often disappears when the drug regimen is changed. But just as clearly, it is too simplistic to blame all impotence on specific drugs.
3. Changes in sleep or dream patterns
4. Positive direct Coombs' test (in 20%) and hemolytic anemia (in 0.2%). Apparently, antibodies to methyldopa cross-react with red cell membranes.
5. Abnormal liver function and hepatitis. Among antihypertensive drugs, this problem is essentially restricted to methyldopa. The mechanism of the liver dysfunction is not understood.
6. Fever. This is a typical "drug fever," caused by obscure mechanisms. It abates quickly when the drug is stopped.
7. Fluid retention (unless diuretics also are given). This is a direct result of reduced arterial pressure (à la Guyton).
8. Dry mouth. This tends to disappear with continued use of the drug. It is a common problem with drugs affecting the sympathetic nervous system.
9. Headache (rare)
10. Postural hypotension and dizziness (uncommon)

Use of Methyldopa in Hypertension

Methyldopa was for a long time the most popular drug to add to diuretics when a second drug was needed to control pressure. It remains an important, dependable, efficacious antihypertensive agent. Central nervous system, hematologic, and hepatic side effects now limit its acceptance. (People with known liver disease should not be given this drug.)

Methyldopa is usually administered orally, 250 mg to 1 gm per dose two times per day. It is nearly *always* used with a diuretic.

Because of its very broad dose–response curve, methyldopa can be used in hypertension of a wide range of severities.

Methyldopa can be given as an injection iv or im, if needed in crisis. It must be infused over a 1-hr period if given iv. By that route, the effectiveness is double that of oral doses.

By whatever route, methyldopa does not exert its full effect until 10–14 days of constant administration. Therefore, doses should not be raised more often than every 2 weeks, unless the pressure is extremely high.

Clonidine (Catapres®)

Mechanism of Action

Clonidine is itself an α-adrenergic agonist; it does not have to be transformed to one. It was originally synthesized to be a nasal vasoconstrictor. It will definitely *constrict* arteries into which it is *infused,* but by the oral route it never reaches a constricting concentration in the arteries.

Clonidine lowers pressure by its actions on a pressure-regulating center in the brain that happens to be α adrenergic. The center's receptors are α_2 in nature. This action is very similar to that of methyldopa.

As a result of altered autonomic nerve traffic, clonidine lowers pressure by a fall in peripheral resistance.

There is no compensatory rise in cardiac rate or output with clonidine, probably because it stimulates α_2 receptors everywhere, and they in turn reduce norepinephrine synthesis.

Renal blood flow is relatively well maintained by clonidine, yet there is a tendency for fluid retention in some patients when the arterial pressure falls significantly. Apparently, the dilation of renal vessels does not fully compensate the glomerulus for the fall in arterial pressure.

Renin release is reduced by clonidine, probably because sympathetic impulses from the brain to the kidney are diminished.

Side Effects

1. Sedation is a very prominent side effect, one which frequently limits acceptance of clonidine by patients.
2. Dry mouth is also a very common side effect; it may abate after several weeks of therapy, but can be very annoying.
3. Fluid retention may result from the reduced head of pressure at the glomerulus caused by clonidine. (Some clinics report surprisingly little fluid retention when clonidine is used alone.)
4. Dizziness can result from reduced pressure and/or sedation.

5. "Rebound" hypertension can occur if the drug is discontinued abruptly from a relatively large dose (1.0 mg or more per day). This is especially common if a β blocker is also being given. The rebound looks like an adrenergic excess, like a pheochromocytoma paroxysm. It can be treated by restarting clonidine or by giving α blockers (e.g., phentolamine).

Use of Clonidine in Hypertension

Clonidine is a "step two" drug of growing popularity, thought of for the same situations as methyldopa. It could be used in place of methyldopa for patients with liver disease.

Clonidine is also becoming popular as a "step four" drug, to be added to a combination of diuretic, β blocker, and vasodilator.

Diuretics potentiate the benefits of clonidine.

Give clonidine orally, 0.1 to 0.2 mg per dose, once or twice a day. Try not to prescribe more than 0.4 mg per day. At higher doses, some vasoconstrictor effect may show up, and rebound hypertension will be a bigger danger, especially when β blockers are also given.

Start giving clonidine in one dose at night, to enable the patient to acclimate to the sedation. Later, give the major part of each day's dose at bedtime, (e.g., 0.1 mg in the morning, and 0.2 mg at night.)

β Blockers make an effective combination with low doses of clonidine, but increase the risk of rebound if the clonidine is stopped. Prazosin (an α blocker) is also a good synergist. It may help prevent rebound.

Clonidine can be useful in cases of sudden, severe elevations of blood pressure. A good example is the hypertension that follows withdrawal of alcohol from an alcoholic. Another example is the hypertension that follows *narcotic withdrawal* (In fact, clonidine reduces other symptoms of narcotic withdrawal, such as sweating, in addition to the hypertension). Presumably, many cases of sudden, severe hypertension are caused by a rush of sympathetic impulses from the brain to the peripheral blood vessels and heart, and clonidine can turn these impulses off. For these cases, give 0.2 mg of clonidine by mouth, and follow with 0.1 mg every hour. Try to avoid giving more than 0.7 mg in any 24-hr period.

17 Drugs Acting on the Autonomic Nervous System: β Blockers

Mechanism of Action*

β Blockers (e.g., propranolol, Inderal) were designed to block the effects of epinephrine on the *heart* and thereby slow it down, make it less irritable, and reduce its strength of contraction to save energy. All β blockers that lower blood pressure have a cardiac effect. However, it is too simplistic to attribute their antihypertensive properties entirely to their ability to slow and soften the heartbeat. Two other effects probably contribute significantly to pressure lowering.

β Blockers *reduce renin release* by the kidneys. Different blockers reduce renin to different degrees. All β blockers on the market today seem to lower

*This is a good time to review Chapter 3.

arterial pressure to roughly the same extent, regardless of their variable ability to lower renin levels in the plasma. A β blocker's ability to lower renin can be useful in treating hypertension (in part by reducing aldosterone secretion and sodium retention as well as by reducing vasoconstriction), but it is certainly not the full explanation for the therapeutic efficacy of these drugs.

Finally, and probably most important, β blockers inhibit *adrenergic pressor centers in the brain.* There are β-adrenergic receptors in the central nervous system that raise peripheral resistance when they are turned on; β blockers turn them off. The result is *lower total peripheral resistance.* It is likely that this effect is the key to the antihypertensive effect of these drugs and may account for the slow achievement of maximum therapeutic effect. (It can take 2 to 4 weeks before the pressure bottoms out on any one dose.)

Side Effects

These are easy to predict if you think of the normal effects of endogenous epinephrine and the benefits epinephrine can accomplish when injected.

1. *Reduced cardiac output,* especially from hearts that are in failure and are driven partly by catecholamines (a β_1 effect)
2. Worsening of preexisting *heart block* (a β_1 effect)
3. Bradycardia, seen in virtually everyone. The resting pulse rate is lowered, and the rise induced by exercise is partially blocked (a β_1 effect).
4. Reduced *exercise tolerance,* seen only in some patients
5. *Bronchospasm,* especially in asthmatics or those with obstructive pulmonary disease whose bronchi are being kept open by endogenous or medicinal catecholamines or sympathomimetic drugs (a β_2 effect).
6. Worsening of *hypoglycemia* in patients receiving insulin or oral hypoglycemics. Normally, when blood glucose falls below a certain level, epinephrine is released from the adrenal medulla. Other hormones such as cortisol, glucagon, and growth hormone also come forth to buffer the falling glucose. Not only is the glycogenolytic effect of epinephrine blocked by β blockers, but also the effects of epinephrine that usually warn the patient that the glucose is low, such as apprehension, tachycardia, and cold skin (β_2 effects).
7. There are some reports of transient high blood potassium levels occurring during exercise, because the ability of catecholamines to drive potassium into cells is blocked.
8. Worsening of *peripheral vascular disease* from unopposed α-adrenergic activity causing vasospasm. The peripheral effects of non-

specific β blockers include blockade of those β receptors that dilate vessels, such as arteries supplying muscle. They are primarily β_2 receptors. When they are blocked, the remaining α effects cause vasoconstriction. This local vasoconstriction usually does not prevent the overall pressure-lowering effects of β blockers, but it can limit the acceptance of the drug in patients with peripheral vascular disease.

9. β Blockers can *aggravate atypical angina* (variant or "Prinzmetal angina"), presumably by the same mechanism that they aggravate peripheral vascular disease—α adrenergic vasoconstriction. This is in sharp contrast to their generally salubrious effects on typical angina. This is discussed further in Chapter 21.
10. β Blockers clearly *affect the brain*. Some of the most annoying side effects are central. Sedation, a sense of listlessness or lack of energy, a general loss of ambition or interest, fatigue, a change in sleep pattern, bad dreams, impotence, and even frank depression can be seen. Women may notice a decreased interest in sex, or reduced vaginal lubrication during sex while on high doses of β blockers or other antihypertensive drugs affecting the nervous system.
11. Note: There is little postural hypotension with these drugs. Apparently, peripheral autonomic reflexes can still maintain acceptable blood pressure by changes in vascular caliber, even though changes in pulse rate are blocked by the drugs. Furthermore, there are little or no bothersome side effects of β blockers on the gut, genitourinary tract, or salivary glands (organs that were badly upset by the older autonomic blocking agents).
12. Finally, there is little fluid retention when β blockers are used alone. Apparently, they have an effect on the kidneys that "encourages" sodium excretion despite a fall in pressure. The nature of this renal effect is unknown, but it is extremely valuable. There is even some evidence that one β blocker (nadolol) increases renal blood flow. It is not absolutely necessary to give diuretics to all patients whose pressure is lowered by β blockers.

Use in Hypertension

β Blockers have become very popular second drugs ("Step two") to add to diuretics when diuretics alone fail to control pressure. β Blockers can also be used alone ("Step one") in selected cases.

These drugs have a smooth, gradual effect with no tolerance appearing, unless fluid retention occurs. In fact, the full antihypertensive effect takes about 2 weeks to develop (although side effects show up more quickly).

These drugs can be used over a broad range of doses (e.g., from 20 to 240 mg of propranolol orally, twice a day). This permits use of β blockers in all hypertensives, from the mildest to the most severe.

β Blockers form a good base of therapy on which to add vasodilators if they are needed as a third drug. The β blockers block the compensatory tachycardia that usually follows use of some vasodilators.

These drugs are especially useful in patients who also have anxiety or a "hyperkinetic" (hyperdynamic) type of hypertension, or other evidence of increased adrenergic activity. These features frequently occur in young patients. In them, β blockers may be sufficient therapy without addition of diuretics. The β blocker may improve the patient's anxiety as well as the hypertension.

β Blockers are particularly useful in patients who also have angina. The reduced cardiac output relieves the pain caused by inadequate coronary flow.

Beware of abruptly discontinuing short-acting β blockers in patients with coronary disease. The rebound of adrenergic stimulation can aggravate angina, cause arrhythmia, or even result in myocardial infarction.

β Blockers may be less effective in patients with hypertension caused by volume expansion than in patients with high cardiac output. This is a relative situation. Although less effective than in hyperdynamic patients, β blockers are still useful in volume-expanded patients. Some clinicians recommend measurement of peripheral renin activity to identify those patients who will do especially well (high renin) or poorly (low renin) on β blockers. This is a vigorously debated issue. High renin levels may well reveal those patients with high endogenous adrenergic activity (renal sympathetic nerves and plasma epinephrine stimulate renin release). Low renin levels may well reveal volume-expanded patients. However, the variability of the measurement is great, and the ability of β blockers to lower pressure is broad. One need not draw renin levels routinely to identify responders to β blockade.

Intravenous doses of β blockers can be unexpectedly potent and toxic, causing cardiac standstill. Use only 1 or 2 mg iv if needed. Give it slowly. This route is only used in treatment of emergencies, such as arrhythmia or aortic dissection.

Because of the side effects listed above, β blockers should *not* be used at all in patients with heart block or heart failure (unless high pressure is causing or aggravating the failure). Care should be exercised whenever β blockers are used in patients with bronchial obstruction or asthma, diabetes treated with insulin or oral hypoglycemic drugs, or in patients with peripheral vascular disease.

New β blockers will stand or fall on the relative number and severity of side effects, because *all of them are effective* at lowering blood pressure in hypertensives.

Choosing among β Blockers

β Blockers that successfully lower blood pressure have proliferated on the market in the past few years. Because they all lower pressure, they must be distinguished from one another by other characteristics. The features that are said to distinguish one β blocker from another are as follows:

1. Selectivity for β_1 (as opposed to β_2) receptors
2. Ability to reduce mortality from myocardial infarction
3. Intrinsic sympathomimetic activity
4. Duration of action
5. Solubility in water or fat solvents
6. Dependability of blood levels as a function of oral dose
7. Membrane stabilization
8. Combined α and β blockade
9. Cost
10. Euphony

Characteristics That Differentiate among β Blockers

Selective Antagonism of β_1 (Cardiac) as Opposed to β_2 (Bronchial and Vasodilator) Receptors

This is a very useful trait among β blockers. Those that can boast of it include metoprolol (Lopressor®) and atenolol (Tenormin®). This trait *may* permit administration of a pressure-lowering dose of β blocker without aggravation of bronchospasm, aggravation of peripheral vascular constriction, or exaggeration of hypoglycemia. Unfortunately, the selectivity is relative, not absolute. Higher doses of the blocker have the same nonspecific effects as nonspecific blockers. Still, these drugs should take precedence over their nonspecific congeners for patients with known bronchospasm, peripheral vascular disease, or hypoglycemic reactions.

Mortality Reduction

The ability to reduce mortality from acute myocardial infarction is a property that has been desired by clinicians since infarction became recognized as a common clinical entity. Since a large proportion of those infarct victims who die from their attack do so in the first two years, and since most of these deaths are attributed to lethal ventricular arrhythmias, it was logical to hope that β blockers would reduce mortality by their antiarrhythmic activity.

Most early trials of β blockers in myocardial infarction yielded equivocal or negative results, until timolol (Blocadren®) was tested in Norway. There, this drug reduced mortality by 25 to 40% during the first 30 months postinfarct. The question immediately arose as to whether this good result represented a fortuitous combination of Nordic physique and novel pharmacology or the first fair and thorough trial of β blockers in a large enough population of infarct victims. Like the four-minute mile, this long-sought achievement in one country was quickly followed by a spate of similar achievements elsewhere. Certainly, protection by β blockers is not reserved for Norwegians. It remained to be seen whether it was as readily achieved by all β blockers as by timolol (Blocadren). A large trial in the United States recently showed significant protection from infarct death by propranolol (Inderal), and the degree of protection was similar to that seen in the Norwegian trial. It is unclear how this protection is achieved. β Blockers not only lower arterial pressure and cardiac work, they affect the conduction system and reduce the tendency of platelets to aggregate. All of these properties might benefit a patient with a fresh, uncomplicated myocardial infarction.

Since these trials are very expensive, we may never know if all β blockers can protect infarct victims. Those companies that have obtained evidence are allowed to crow about it (and they *are* crowing). Protection of infarct victims represents a huge potential bonus for β blockers in hypertension. After all, it is to reduce cardiovascular complications that we lower high blood pressure in the first place. If a given treatment not only slows atherosclerosis by lowering pressure, but also protects from its complications, it would be a treatment easy to recommend (and risky to omit).

Two things prevent the clinician from prescribing a β blocker to everyone with hypertension: undesirable side effects that may outweigh its value to patients who are not prone to heart attacks (e.g., young patients and women); and the lingering doubts of efficacy in myocardial infarction left by early failures to demonstrate protection. Perhaps benefits are restricted to patients with recent infarcts and no complications. For example, there is clearly some risk in giving β blockers to those with conduction defects or failure.

Intrinsic Sympathomimetic Activity (ISA)

This is a property that seems paradoxical in a β-blocker. It means that the blocker partially overcomes its own blockade. This feature permits β blockade with less bradycardia, perhaps less tendency to heart failure, perhaps less bronchoconstriction, and perhaps less "rebound" if and when the drug is discontinued. Intrinsic sympathomimetic activity also helps prevent overtreatment. There is a predetermined ratio of agonism-to-antagonism (antidote-to-antagonist) in each tablet. Apparently, the epinephrine-like activity does not lessen the ability of these β-blockers to lower blood pressure. The blocking activity lowers pressure whereas the epinephrine-like activity helps sustain heart rate, cardiac contractility, bronchodilation, and receptor "down-regulation."

Receptor down-regulation is the lowering of responsiveness in a target by a hormone. Normally, epinephrine holds down the number of its own receptors, keeping targets relatively unresponsive. In its absence or in the case of antagonism by blockers, targets become hyperresponsive to epinephrine. (Remember denervation hypersensitivity?) β Blockers block down-regulation and lead to hypersensitivity to catecholamines. Discontinuation of β blockers leads to "rebound" responsiveness to intrinsic epinephrine and to angina or arrhythmias in some patients. β Blockers with sympathomimetic activity keep epinephrine receptors down-regulated, keep targets from becoming hypersensitive, and presumably can be stopped suddenly with greater safety.

In general, the advantage gained from the use of β blockers with intrinsic sympathomimetic activity pertains most directly to patients with heart disease. This property recommends their use in patients with unusually slow pulse rates. It remains to be proven whether side effects on the bronchi and peripheral arteries can be better avoided by using selective blockers or by drugs with an intrinsic combination of agonist and antagonist activity.

Prolonged Duration of Action

This is characteristic of some β blockers, notably nadolol (Corgard®), atenolol (Tenormin), timolol (Blocadren) and the newest, carteolol. These can be taken once a day with no sacrifice in efficacy. This is an advantage to patients who tend to forget medicines during the day; but experience has shown that even the short-acting β blockers such as propranolol effectively lower blood pressure when taken only twice a day. (The same may *not* be true for their ability to relieve angina or tachy-arrhythmias). Long-acting β blockers can more easily accumulate to dangerous levels in patients with renal failure, so longevity is not an unmixed blessing.

Solubility in Water versus Lipids (Hydrophilicity versus Lipophilicity)

This is a physicochemical property of β blockers that is easy to measure in the laboratory. It is a property that also affects the mechanism by which drugs are excreted or inactivated—water-soluble drugs are excreted primarily in the urine, lipid-soluble drugs are usually conjugated in the liver before being excreted. Thus, hydrophilic drugs are more susceptible to accumulation in renal failure, and lipophilic ones tend to accumulate in hepatic failure. Among β blockers, the long-acting ones are more water soluble.

It seems logical, but is not proven, that lipid-soluble drugs cross into the brain more readily than water-soluble ones, and exert more psychotropic side effects. (It might also be true that lipid-soluble drugs more readily block the nervous centers that elevate pressure.) We do not know the relevance of solubility to the therapeutic : toxic ratio (the "bottom line" in all drug comparisons). Solubility is a reproducible parameter of drugs perhaps best ignored until its relevance is known.

Dependability of Blood Levels with a Prescribed Oral Dose

This is a useful property for any drug. The duration of action of those β blockers that are inactivated primarily by hepatic metabolism is difficult to predict. The liver is altered by many drugs, by alcohol, by passive congestion, etc. Each change affects the ability of the liver to inactivate drugs such as β blockers. This has been a problem endured by propranolol (Inderal) since its invention.

When hepatic inactivation is extensive, a large proportion of an oral dose can be lost between absorption into the portal circulation and arrival in the vena cava. This is called the "First Pass" effect—referring to the drug's interactions during its first passage through the liver. By contrast, longer-acting β blockers such as nadolol (Corgard), timolol (Blocadren), and atenolol (Tenormin) are relatively immune to hepatic inactivation. They are inactivated in the kidneys, a more predictable organ than the liver. Thus, the blood levels achieved by long-acting β blockers bear a more reliable relationship to the oral dose from patient to patient and from day to day.

The last three qualities of β blockers can be lumped together: duration of action, water solubility, and dependability of blood levels. They are related and tend to track together.

Membrane Stabilization

This is an effect best shown by propranolol (Inderal). It can be thought of as a kind of local anesthesia at the cellular level, and it may have some relevance when heroic doses of drug are used. Many effective β blockers do not have this property, so membrane stabilization can be safely ignored until its importance is demonstrated.

Combined Antagonism of α and β Receptors

This property is intellectually appealing in an antihypertensive. One drug has it (labetalol). It is used overseas, but not yet in the United States. This drug is a more potent antihypertensive than pure β blockers. It has one predictable shortcoming that other β blockers avoid: inhibition of the vasoconstrictor limb of postural reflexes. Postural hypotension can be a problem for patients on this drug, as for those taking prazosin, a pure α blocker. The fixed ratio of α and β blockade in labetolol makes it impossible to titrate the two activities separately in individual patients. The niche for this drug is uncertain, but there is no doubt that it is a novel and efficacious agent.

The Financial Cost of Medication

Cost becomes a highly significant variable when one considers the lifelong duration of hypertension treatment. Makers of older or nonpatented drugs tend to protect their market from flashy newcomers by slashing prices. The least costly β blocker is the oldest, propranolol (Inderal). The most expensive ones cost three times more for equivalent doses.

Two factors mitigate the cost issue: (1) savings can be realized by using agents that permit fewer tablets at longer intervals and (2) people with good health insurance or good Dun and Bradstreet ratings tend to be relatively oblivious to cost. At the least, cost is a quality of β blockers that the most naive patient or practitioner can measure and compare.

Euphony

Euphony refers to the sound of the name of the drug. The ease with which the name trips off the tongue, and the clues it gives to the drug's effect, are not only esthetically appealing, but can be an adjunct to therapy.

The clumsy suffix ''olol'' in the generic name tells us that we are dealing with a β blocker. (In case there is any residual ambiguity, ''Blocadren'' makes things quite explicit.) This information might prevent the *clinician* from prescribing two drugs with the same effect to the same patient. By the

TABLE I

Distinguishing Characteristics of β Blockers

Selectivity for β_1	*Protection from infarct mortality*	*Intrinsic sympathomimetic activity*	*Long acting*	*Combined α and β blockade*	*Low cost*
Metoprolol	Timolol	Pindolol	Nadolol	Labetolol	Propranolol
Atenolol	Propranolol	Carteolol	Atenolol		
	(Metoprolol)[a]	Oxprenolol	Timolol		
	(Atenolol)[a]		Carteolol		

[a] Small studies yielded suggestive results.

same token, Lopressor and Corgard help inform the *patient* of the goal of the treatment and help the physician communicate by talking about the "heart pill" or the "pressure medicine." Combined with a distinctive shape, color, or decoration, an effective name can be a boon to compliance. Politicians and movie moguls have used these tricks for generations.

Table I (p. 145) lists some marketed and investigational β blockers according to the special characteristics listed above.

Drug Interactions

β Blockers have a predictable interaction with sympathomimetic drugs, such as isoproterenol, epinephrine, and nasal vasoconstrictors. In the presence of β blockers, these drugs exert much less of an effect on the heart and bronchi. On the other hand, β blockers exaggerate the pressor, peripheral vasoconstrictor effects of these substances, and a dramatic rise in arterial pressure may occur as a result of this interaction.

β Blockers can have a negative inotropic effect, reducing the strength of cardiac contraction as a result of diminished effects of endogenous catecholamines. Another group of drugs with negative inotropic effects are the *calcium channel blocking agents*. When β blockers and calcium channel blockers are used simultaneously, there may be a dangerous drop in cardiac output in some patients. This is more likely to be a problem with verapamil than with nifedipine. Calcium channel blockers should be used with caution in patients who also receive β blockers.

18 Other Antihypertensive Drugs That Affect the Nervous System

Reserpine (A Rauwolfia Alkaloid)

Mechanism of Action

Reserpine *blocks nerve cell uptake and storage* of catecholamines, depletes the nerves of their transmitter, thereby resulting in smaller releases of NE from firing cells in both the CNS and the peripheral autonomic system.

The circulatory result of reduced autonomic activity is reduced peripheral resistance and reduced cardiac output. The pulse rate slows.

Because cardiovascular reflexes are intact, there is little or no postural hypotension with reserpine.

Reserpine reduces renin release by the kidneys.

Side Effects

1. Reserpine is notorious for causing psychiatric depression, which can lead to suicide. This must obviously be considered a truly fatal poten-

tial side effect. The incidence of this side effect is significant only at doses over 0.5 mg per day. To be safe, most clinicians recommend much less. In fact good pressure control can be attained with as little as 0.1 mg of reserpine every other day combined with a diuretic.

2. Reserpine is a good tranquilizer. It ushered in a whole era (The Road to Miltown), but is not used much in psychiatry today.
3. "Stuffy nose" is very common with reserpine. This is a consequence of unopposed parasympathetic activity. (The opposite of the clear nose one gets from a squirt of sympathomimetic nose spray.)
4. Gastrointestinal side effects of reserpine include nausea, increased acid secretion, symptoms of peptic ulcer, and diarrhea, all from unopposed parasympathetic activity.
5. Bradycardia and reduced cardiac output can be considered reserpine side effects as well as part of its mechanism of action. When used with a vasodilator like hydralazine, reserpine's ability to slow the pulse is an advantage.
6. Reserpine can cause a syndrome indistinguishable from Parkinson's disease. Parkinsonism is the result of extreme depletion of catecholamines from the basal ganglia of the brain. Observation of this side effect, and its interpretation by Dr. J. Axelrod, led to the development of therapy with dopa to replenish catecholamines in brains of patients with idiopathic Parkinsonism.
7. There are conflicting reports about a possible relationship between the use of reserpine and the development of breast cancer. Although the maximum number of cancers theoretically caused by reserpine is very low, any possible relationship is frightening. This suggests caution in the use of the drug in women with a history suggesting higher than normal cancer risk, such as a family history of breast cancer.
8. There are some classical *drug interactions* with reserpine. Since it depletes neuronal catecholamines, it *blocks* the effects of *indirect* adrenergic drugs such as ephedrine and amphetamine. (Those drugs work by releasing stored catecholamines.) Because it blocks uptake of catecholamines by cells that could degrade them, it *potentiates* the action of *direct* adrenergic agents such as norepinephrine and of monamine oxidase (MAO) inhibitors.

Use of Reserpine in Hypertension

Reserpine has a slow, smooth onset of hypotensive action, reaching maximum in 4–6 weeks.

It is almost always effective, but its effect is not great, especially since it is necessary to keep the dose low to minimize sedation and depression. Therefore, reserpine is not commonly used in severe hypertension. However, when used with a diuretic, reserpine can be very valuable in the management of some patients. It also can prevent the tachycardia that would otherwise accompany use of vasodilators.

Typical reserpine doses range from 0.05 to 0.25 mg per day by mouth in one dose. The drug has a long duration of action. It can also be given by injection in emergencies.

Despite its unfortunate reputation, this drug refuses to die. It is so gentle and smooth in its hypotensive action that its convenience and low price often outweigh fears of depression and cancer.

It is a safe, conservative rule *never* to use reserpine in a patient with a past history or family history of depression or breast cancer or with any condition that might lead to either of these (e.g., divorce, bereavement, cystic mastitis). It is also dangerous to use reserpine in patients with untreated peptic ulcer.

Guanethidine (Ismelin®)

Mechanism of Action

Guanethidine *blocks release* of norepinephrine by nerves, and also depletes those nerves of catecholamines.

Guanethidine acts only peripherally. *It does not cross into the brain*. Therefore, it has no direct central nervous system side effects!

Guanethidine lowers peripheral resistance and reduces cardiac output. It does NOT open up renal vessels. In fact, renal blood flow decreases with typical doses of guanethidine. Therefore, fluid retention frequently complicates its use.

Guanethidine must be taken into the nerves before it lowers pressure; this is achieved by the same pump that takes up norepinephrine. Therefore, blockers of this pump block guanethidine action. The norepinephrine pump blockers include tricyclic antidepressants. Thus, tricyclics block the beneficial effects of guanethidine. (This is probably the most thoroughly documented *drug interaction* known to man. Its discovery was seminal to the birth of the field now known as clinical pharmacology.)

Side Effects

1. *Postural hypotension* is a real problem with guanethidine. The sudden pressure drop causes serious problems in the heads and hearts of people with vascular insufficiency.
2. Fluid retention is fairly common when guanethidine lowers arterial pressure (unless diuretics are also used).

3. Diarrhea from unopposed parasympathetic activity can be a very troublesome side effect.
4. Retrograde ejaculation, failure of ejaculation, or impotence can complicate guanethidine therapy. Sex is, after all, nothing less than an expression of the vegetative nervous system at its best. (It may be more, but never less.) Almost all drugs affecting the autonomic nervous system affect sexual functions in males. Effects on females are less well recognized, or less vividly reported, or just less frequent. (By contrast, retrograde ejaculation, wherein semen is forced back into the bladder, is very vivid.)
5. The first dose of guanethidine may cause a transient release of catecholamines, with a concomitant burst of hypertension. When a pheochromocytoma is present, this can be more a blast than a burst. Although dangerous, this is a helpful hint that a pheochromocytoma exists.
6. By depleting cardiac catecholamines, guanethidine can reduce cardiac output, especially in patients with failing hearts that are partially "driven" by endogenous catecholamines. As in the case of β blockers, this reduction in cardiac output can be dangerous.

Use in Hypertension

Guanethidine is a "big gun," used currently in severe hypertension only.

Guanethidine has a slow onset and a slow decay. One should change doses weekly or biweekly only. After the drug is stopped, its effects may last for weeks.

Give guanethidine orally in doses of from 10 to 300 mg, only once per day.

Use guanethidine with diuretics. They will block its tendency to cause fluid retention and will markedly potentiate its effectiveness.

Attend to the postural hypotension problem. Pressure lowering by guanethidine is largely the result of pooling of blood in the legs when a patient stands up. Because so much of the hypotensive effect is postural, a patient's pressure can rise dramatically when he/she lies down and sends pooled blood back into the central circulation. Patients may need to use blocks under the heads of their beds to maintain a semiupright posture at night.

Avoid guanethidine in ambulatory patients with cerebral insufficiency or coronary insufficiency. The fluctuations in pressure with posture and exercise are poorly tolerated by ischemic brains and hearts!

Bethanidine

This is a new congener of guanethidine. It has a shorter duration of action and is reported to cause less diarrhea. We must wait to see if these improvements will enable more widespread use of bethanidine than guanethidine. Until proven otherwise, both of these drugs seem destined for use only in patients with very resistant hypertension.

Effects Common to Drugs Acting on the Nervous System

Except for guanethidine, all drugs that affect the autonomic nervous system reduce plasma renin levels.

Except for guanethidine and prazosin, these drugs cause very little postural hypotension.

All drugs of this class, except guanethidine and prazosin, can cause changes in the psyche: either bad dreams, sexual dysfunction, sedation, lethargy, lack of "energy," or frank depression.

Other side effects of drugs acting on the nervous system read like a list of autonomic malfunctions: bradycardia, dry mouth, diarrhea, peptic ulcer, stuffy nose, impotence, retrograde ejaculation, etc. Not all drugs have the complete list of dysfunctions, but all have some.

19 Vasodilators, Converting-Enzyme Inhibitors, and Angiotensin Blockers

Introduction

Whatever the initial stimulus to high arterial blood pressure, the final effectors that achieve pressure elevation are the heart and the resistance vessels (BP = CO × TPR). Of these two, the peripheral resistance vessels are more reasonable targets to "attack" or modify in treatment. (It seems obviously more dangerous to tamper with the heart.) Furthermore, established hypertension in adults is characterized by increased peripheral resistance, not increased cardiac output. Apparently, the vessels in chronic hypertension develop thicker walls or greater contractility. Thus, it is not only safer, but more logical to treat the vessels instead of the heart, especially in long-standing hypertension.

Because the heart and peripheral arteries are also the final mediators of *cardiovascular reflexes,* drugs that affect these organs make patients more vulnerable to precipitous drops in pressure during changes in posture or exercise. (This is in contrast to drugs acting on pressure-integrating centers in the brain. They can lower the pressure set-point without blunting rapid reflexes.) The drugs described in this chapter affect vascular smooth muscle directly or the pressor agents that cause vascular constriction. They are, as a class, the most easily rationalized hypotensive agents.

Hydralazine (Apresoline®)

Mechanism of Action

Hydralazine directly relaxes vascular smooth muscle by a mildly toxic effect on the contractile machinery (not the membrane). Hydralazine has its greatest effect on vessels supplying the viscera, including the renal vessels. There is relatively little effect on vessels supplying skin or muscle.

Thanks to a dilating effect on renal vasculature, hydralazine preserves renal blood flow and renal function despite a fall in systemic pressure. This is a very valuable property for an antihypertensive drug. Without it, the fall in pressure in the renal artery would reduce glomerular filtration and lead to fluid retention. By dilating renal vessels, hydralazine tends to compensate for the reduced head of pressure, passing more of the arterial pressure on to the glomerulus.

Part of the vasodilating action of hydralazine is apparently mediated by prostaglandin release, because the drug is less effective when given with nonsteroidal antiinflammatory drugs (NSAIDs) like indomethacin (Indocin®) or ibuprofen (Motrin®). These drugs block prostaglandin synthesis and reduce the effectiveness of many antihypertensive agents.

Hydralazine causes *cardiac reflexes* to kick in, resulting in *tachycardia* and *increased cardiac output* when the drug lowers arterial pressure.

Tachycardia is the only response that the *cardiovascular* system can invoke in its attempt to restore pressure to its pretreatment level (since the treatment itself blocks the other cardiovascular response—vasoconstriction.) *Renin re-*

lease occurs when a vasodilator lowers arterial pressure. This is the standard endocrine response to abrupt falls in pressure. The autonomic nervous system also responds with release of catecholamines from the adrenal medulla. Both plasma renin and plasma catecholamine levels rise during hydralazine therapy, but not enough to keep the pressure up. These changes contribute to fluid retention and tachycardia, however.

Side Effects

1. *Tachycardia* and palpitations are common when hydralazine is used alone.
2. If the coronary circulation is compromised, angina pectoris can be aggravated by hydralazine. The occurrence of this side effect depends on the net effect of vasodilation to lower pressure and compensatory reflexes to cause tachycardia. Lowered pressure *spares* the heart some of its work and oxygen requirements. Tachycardia (increased output) *costs* the heart more work and oxygen. In general, pressure-work is more expensive than output-work, so lowered pressure generally spares the heart despite an increased pulse rate. If reflex tachycardia does *not* occur, vasodilators exert a purely beneficial effect on a heart starved for oxygen and substrates. (This line of reasoning is the basis for treating intractable heart failure by vasodilators, the so-called *afterload reduction* therapy.)
3. An inflammatory disease resembling *lupus erythematosus*—with fever, arthritis, and LE cells—is seen in some patients when doses of hydralazine exceed 300 mg per day. It is primarily seen among "slow acetylators," people whose livers inactivate the drug slowly. (Unfortunately, a patient's acetylation capacity is never known in advance.)
4. Hydralazine can cause a throbbing *headache* as a result of dilation of the arteries supplying the head and the usual increase in cardiac output and blood flow.

Use in Hypertension

Hydralazine is most logically used as a "Step 3" drug, to be added if a diuretic plus an autonomic blocker or CNS drug fail to control the pressure.

Simultaneous use of a β blocker prevents tachycardia and headache and augments the usefulness of hydralazine. (If a β blocker is contraindicated, some of the same benefits can be obtained from methyldopa, clonidine, or reserpine.)

Hydralazine can be used as a "Step 2" drug if tachycardia is not a problem. (Many older patients have blunted baroreceptor reflexes and do not have much tachycardia with hydralazine.)

Give hydralazine orally or by injection. Orally, 25–100 mg per dose two times a day is common.

Hydralazine is probably the fastest acting and fastest decaying of the common antihypertensive drugs. This makes it useful in treating short-term events such as postoperative hypertension. For these situations, the intramuscular route is useful.

Although cardiac side effects and headache are greatly reduced by giving hydralazine with a β blocker or reserpine, *the lupus-like syndrome* is not prevented by the combination. (Of course, addition of a β blocker usually reduces the dose needed for control of pressure.) To be safe, many people consider 200 mg per day as the maximum dose. A higher dose is tolerated by people who acetylate drugs rapidly. However, if "acetylator status" is not known, stay below the 200 mg per day ceiling.

Always try to use a diuretic with hydralazine. Diuretics potentiate the efficacy of vasodilators, and diuretics prevent the fluid retention that may accompany a fall in pressure.

Because it dilates renal vessels, hydralazine is valuable in patients with impaired renal function (e.g., those who display a rise in BUN or creatinine when their pressures fall).

Remember the negative effect of nonsteroidal antiinflammatory drugs on the efficacy of hydralazine and other vasodilators.

Use in Heart Failure

Because it opens up arterioles, hydralazine lowers afterload, the major determinant of cardiac metabolism. In patients with weak myocardium or narrow coronaries, this effect can be useful. However, there is always the potential danger that an excessive fall in diastolic pressure will lower coronary blood flow more than it lowers cardiac metabolism or that tachycardia will make excessive demands. This therapy requires care.

Other vasodilators, such as captopril and prazosin, are also used to achieve afterload reduction in heart failure, and they have the advantage over hydralazine of causing less tachycardia. Most cardiologists consider afterload reduction as a therapeutic modality in all *intractable* cases of cardiac failure, and *try it early when arterial pressure is elevated*. When *preload* reduction is also needed (reduced venous return to the heart) an agent like nitroprusside is more suitable than those mentioned above. It dilates veins and arteries.

Minoxidil (Loniten®)

Mechanism of Action

Minoxidil, like hydralazine, is a vasodilator with a direct effect on smooth muscle in the vessel wall.

Unlike hydralazine, minoxidil does not have a selective vasodilating effect on renal vessels. Therefore, renal blood flow can fall when the pressure drops.

Renin release is stimulated by minoxidil (as is true of all vasodilators except prazosin).

Side Effects

1. Fluid retention almost always occurs when minoxidil lowers the pressure. (Note the difference between this and hydralazine.) This can lead to weight gain, edema, and even pulmonary congestion. The retention can be very severe, necessitating heroic doses of loop diuretics.
2. Tachycardia is stimulated by minoxidil.
3. Growth of unwanted hair in females (or unneeded hair in males) is a common side effect of minoxidil. This affects the face and virtually every other follicle-bearing surface. The company producing this drug is trying a topical form for balding men in an attempt to "capitalize" on the side effect. (In this case, what's gross on a goose looks great on a gander.)

Use in Hypertension

Currently, minoxidil is used in severe hypertensives only, as a "Step 3" or "Step 4" drug. It is thought of as a more potent hydralazine-like drug, used when hydralazine fails or its use is feared because of the lupus-like syndrome.

Minoxidil must be given with a diuretic, usually a potent loop diuretic such as furosemide (Lasix), to overcome its associated fluid retention. A β blocker is also useful in preventing reflex tachycardia.

Minoxidil can be given twice a day, at oral doses of from 2 to 40 mg.

Although it causes sodium retention, minoxidil will preserve renal excretory function if it successfully lowers pressure. In other words, sodium may be retained, but the serum creatinine excretion may improve. (This protection of renal function is a property of *all* successful antihypertensive drugs, even though they cause specific alterations in some renal functions. It is most marked in severe hypertension or in the presence of diabetes.)

Nitroprusside (Nipride®)

Mechanism of Action

Nitroprusside is a potent agent that directly relaxes most smooth muscles, including those in arteries and veins.

Because it dilates veins as well as arteries, nitroprusside does *not* cause compensatory tachycardia or increased cardiac output. (No venous return, no cardiac response!)

Nitroprusside should lower the pressure of every living organism with a pressure to lower. (If it seems to be failing, check the manometer to make sure it is not stuck!)

Side Effects

1. There is a dramatic postural effect with this potent vasodilator, and if dosage is not monitored, fatal hypotension can result whether the patient is standing or lying down.
2. Nitroprusside is first metabolized to cyanide, then to thiocyanate in the liver. Side effects relate to all three agents: the intact drug, cyanide, and thiocyanate.
3. Cyanide formed from nitroprusside can cause death from cerebral or myocardial failure. Fortunately, hydroxycobalamin (vitamin B_{12a}) is a good antidote to cyanide and can be given with nitroprusside. Hydroxycobalamin comes in 10-mg vials and should be infused over several hours. It scavenges cyanide mole for mole. Most people use it after cyanide poisoning has become apparent. It also makes sense as prophylaxis.
4. Thiocyanate formed from nitroprusside blocks iodine uptake by the thyroid and can lead to hypothyroidism. This is only relevant in long-term use of the drug.
5. The most common side effects of nitroprusside are nausea, restlessness, and abdominal cramps. It is not known which chemical species causes these.

Use in Hypertension

Nitroprusside must be given iv, from a bottle wrapped in foil to keep out light and retard decomposition of the drug. It has an extremely rapid onset and decay of activity. As discussed in Chapter 22, nitroprusside is the drug of choice for rapid, guaranteed pressure reduction in a crisis situation or in the operating room, when careful monitoring is available.

Use in Heart Failure

Because it dilates arteries, nitroprusside reduces the afterload of the heart. Because it dilates veins, nitroprusside reduces preload. (Preload is the load of blood entering the heart demanding ejection.) Taken together, these properties make nitroprusside an excellent agent for emergency treatment of refractory cardiac failure. Its action on veins makes nitroprusside especially useful. In patients with evidence of excessive venous pressure, nitroprusside (and vigorous diuresis) may be preferable to use of pure arterial dilators. On the other hand, in patients with very low venous pressure, nitroprusside's action on veins may make matters worse by reducing cardiac output. Patients in severe heart failure require individualized care.

Diazoxide (Hyperstat®)

Mechanism of Action

Although diazoxide is chemically related to the thiazide diuretics, it has no diuretic effect. Instead, it causes quickly what the thiazides cause slowly—arterial vasodilatation. (This fact encourages the belief that ordinary thiazide diuretics truly have an arterial site of action on blood pressure in addition to their effect on the kidneys.)

Diazoxide directly relaxes vascular smooth muscle, primarily in arteries, less in veins, and to some extent in the uterus. It probably exerts its effects on smooth muscle cells by blocking calcium channels in the membrane.

Side Effects

1. Tachycardia and increased cardiac output follow administration of diazoxide.
2. Fluid retention of major proportions follows use of diazoxide. (It may be a *thiazide* but it *is not* a *diuretic!*)
3. Postural hypotension is a constant accompaniment of diazoxide use.
4. High blood glucose levels can be a problem if diazoxide is used for more than a few days. Insulin secretion is blocked by the drug. This is an exaggeration of the hyperglycemic effect seen after thiazide diuretics. (In fact, this effect occasioned the first approved use of diazoxide—to support the blood sugar in patients with hypoglycemia.)
5. Although pressures tend to bottom out at 120/80, an excessive fall in pressure can be caused by too much diazoxide. The bolus form of administration leaves little room for any reaction by the clinician other

than a whispered "whoops" and a hurried move to elevate the patient's legs.

6. Diazoxide inhibits contraction of other smooth muscles, so it causes inhibition of uterine contractions during labor.

Use in Hypertension

After infusion of diazoxide, arterial pressure falls within minutes. It rarely falls below 120/80 (unlike the effects of nitroprusside). It almost appears that diazoxide lyses the "hypertensive" part of the blood pressure, leaving only the "normal" part!

Currently, diazoxide is only given iv in *crisis* situations. Because the reflex tachycardia it causes increases cardiac output, it is *not* used in dissecting aneurysm of the aorta (see Chapter 22).

Because the pressure remains low after the drug has been given, and the needle withdrawn, diazoxide is better than nitroprusside in situations where constant pressure monitoring is a problem. In general, diazoxide is a less certain but safer hypotensive agent than nitroprusside.

Because it is extremely tightly bound to albumin, diazoxide must be given *intravenously very rapidly,* in a bolus of 60–300 mg. When infused as a bolus, some of the drug binds to nearby albumin molecules and some stays free to interact with smooth muscle cells as the blood whips around the circulation. (If the drug is dribbled in, *all* of it is sucked up by the albumin.)

Doses of 60 mg or more can be repeated as needed in repeated iv boluses, but effectiveness wanes in 2 to 3 days. Now that people are using frequent, small boluses instead of a whole vial, excessive hypotension is less common than when it was given in 300 mg slugs.

A diuretic such as furosemide should be given simultaneously to overcome the fluid retention that follows diazoxide use, and a β blocker is also a good idea to overcome tachycardia.

Converting-Enzyme Inhibitors

Mechanism of Action

Drugs [*such as captopril* (*Capoten®*)], that block angiotensin converting enzyme (ACE), mimick vasodilators in many ways, and so they are listed in this chapter. However, these new agents are a dramatic conceptual departure in hypertension therapy. *They reduce formation of the vasoconstrictor angiotensin and prolong the lifespan of the vasodilator bradykinin.* Both effects dilate blood vessels susceptible to these polypeptides. (In addition, ACE can cleave enkephalins, the endogenous opioids. We do not yet know if preservation of enkephalins is relevant to captopril's actions.)

The effect of ACE blockers on blood pressure depends on the activity of the renin–angiotensin and kallikrein–kinin systems. If renin activity is low, blocking it will be unimportant. If kallikrein activity is low, there will not be much bradykinin to protect. There are patients with high renin activity caused by renal disease or stimulation of renin release by catecholamines. These are obvious candidates for captopril treatment. In addition, almost all patients treated by salt restriction, diuretics, or vasodilators develop high renin levels as part of the body's defenses against pressure drops. As a result of stimulated renin release, these patients also become susceptible to the pressure-lowering action of captopril. Thus, an ACE inhibitor may sooner or later become valuable as a hypotensive drug in almost all patients, whatever their *initial* renin level.

ACE inhibitors have dilating effects on *renal* vessels, promoting excretion of sodium in patients who tend to retain it because of low renal blood flow. This effect on renal vessels can be a great boon to antihypertensive therapy.

Part of the antihypertensive action of ACE inhibitors results from prostaglandin release (perhaps caused by increased levels of bradykinin). Simultaneous administration of nonsteroidal antiinflammatory drugs like indomethacin or aspirin reduces the efficacy of drugs like captopril.

Side Effects of Captopril

1. A maculopapular rash, frequently accompanied by fever, occurs in about 5% of patients taking captopril. This may reverse spontaneously despite continued use of the drug. However, most people who experience this side effect stop the drug.
2. An unusual taste or a lack of taste perception ("dysgeusia") is fairly common at the start of captopril therapy. This too, usually disappears after a few weeks of continuous use.
3. Proteinuria is a rare (1%) side effect of captopril that usually occurs in patients who have slight proteinuria or known renal disease before therapy. It is a side effect that should be monitored. If proteinuria continues or progresses, switch to other drugs.
4. Marrow suppression, especially leukopenia, is the most worrisome side effect of captopril. This effect *reverses upon cessation of the drug* (unlike the often-irreversible marrow suppression with chloramphenicol). It occurs in about 1 in 1000 patients taking captopril, and a higher proportion of those with severe complications of hypertension, such as renal impairment. Although marrow depression

caused by captopril is reversible, fatal infections that arise during marrow depression are not. The white count must be monitored!

5. Dramatic drops in blood pressure can be seen in patients taking captopril. This is just another manifestation of its great efficacy in some patients.
6. Captopril causes fetal death in rabbits. Do *not* use it in pregnant women.
7. Although converting-enzyme inhibitors raise plasma renin activity, the peptide cascade started by renin only gets as far as angiotensin I.

Note how *few* of the typical side effects of antihypertensive drugs ACE inhibitors exert:

They do *not* cause hypokalemia, hyperuricemia, or hyperglycemia.

They do *not* cause sedation, depression, or sexual dysfunction.

They do *not* cause headache, lupus, angina, fluid retention, bradycardia, heart block, tachycardia, or heart failure.

Use in Hypertension and Heart Failure

Captopril was initially recommended solely for cases of hypertension poorly controlled on traditional therapy. It soon became apparent that the drug was effective in patients with mild as well as severe hypertension. Although it works best in those patients with high plasma renin activity, it works reasonably well in *most* patients. Apparently, a large proportion of hypertensives obtain some degree of blood pressure support from the renin–angiotensin–aldosterone system. (The same can be said for the sympathetic nervous system: it can be attacked by drugs, resulting in therapeutic benefits, despite the fact that all known parameters of its activity are normal.)

Captopril and its successors should ultimately become ideal "Step Two" drugs. They antagonize the compensatory rise in renin that impedes full effectiveness of Step One diuretics. A diuretic plus an ACE inhibitor is a very sensible combination, and has *no* CNS side effects.

Captopril alone successfully normalizes pressure in about 30% of mild hypertensives. It, or less toxic successors, may some day rival diuretics as initial therapy for the average patient.

Captopril has unique effectiveness in *scleroderma renal disease*. It is life-saving there. It also works in some cases of *primary pulmonary hypertension*.

Captopril dilates veins as well as arteries and is an ideal drug to treat refractory heart failure by a combination of *afterload reduction, preload reduction,* and even some *coronary vasodilation!*

A typical dose of captopril is 50 mg two or three times per day, by mouth.

Some people respond to 25 mg b.i.d. The maximum dose is 150 t.i.d. *Dosage should be halved for patients with renal impairment.*

It is best to take captopril on an empty stomach. Food and antacids retard its absorption.

Newer ACE Inhibitors

One new ACE inhibitor (Enalapril) is close to release, and others are in the pipeline. It will be interesting to see their side effect spectrum. It is unlikely that new ones will be more efficacious than captopril, but they may cause fewer side effects. If they do not cause marrow suppression, rash, fever, or proteinuria, they will be welcome additions to antihypertensive therapy.

Saralasin (Pronounced "Sa-rá-lazin", or "Sarah Layzin") (Sarenin®)

This peptide analog of angiotensin (*sar*cosine in position 1, *ala*nine in position 8) antagonizes angiotensin at its receptor.

The drug has some angiotensin-like activity. It is not a pure antagonist. This situation is called "partial agonism." (It caused a good deal of "agony" in the company that manufactures the drug.) Partial agonism results in a burst of increased pressure when the drug is started in patients with low renin levels.

Because it is a peptide, this drug must be given iv and not po.

Saralasin probably will *not* make a big impact on treatment, except in people with malignant hypertension who cannot take captopril. It may be useful in diagnosis of high renin states. In this respect, it is analogous to phentolamine (Regitine®) which is used to diagnose states with increased catecholamine production.

Prazosin

This drug was described in Chapter 16 on autonomic antagonists. It is an α adrenergic blocker. However, it can be thought of as a vasodilator and can be used in therapy before more potent vasodilators are invoked. Its action on α receptors causes arterial vasodilation. Because prazosin does not block α_2 receptors, synthesis of norepinephrine remains repressed by negative feedback via presynaptic α_2 receptors. The reduced norepinephrine synthesis lessens "overflow" of catecholamines in the circulation, and tachycardia is *not* a problem when this drug successfully lowers pressure.

Effects Common to Vasodilators

The biggest worry with the use of vasodilators is postural hypotension. The normal reflex response to a drop in pressure includes vasoconstriction. Vasodilators impede that crucial compensation.

All vasododilators except prazosin stimulate release of renin from the kidneys.

Most vasodilators cause reflex tachycardia and can cause angina or pounding headaches in susceptible patients. This is not a problem with prazosin or captopril and less of a problem with nitroprusside.

Although elderly patients may suffer the consequences of tachycardia more than young ones, they are mercifully less susceptible to the tachycardia itself. Apparently, their baroreceptor reflexes age along with their arteries.

Current practice favors concomitant use of β blockers along with the pure vasodilators such as hydralazine and minoxidil when tachycardia is potentially dangerous (as in people with known coronary artery insufficiency).

20 Drug Combinations, Drug Resistance, and Drug Selection

Introduction

Traditional pharmacologic teaching dictates that diseases be treated with as few drugs as possible, in doses as low as possible. Although this is sound advice for diseases in which the cause is known, like infection, it does not make as much sense in the treatment of hypertension. In hypertension, *none* of the drugs actually treat the underlying *cause* of the disorder. In most cases, the cause is unknown.

Drugs used in hypertension attack one or more *normal* physiological processes that support blood pressure. There are many mechanisms that support blood pressure, and we do not know which, if any, are abnormal in patients. Furthermore, many of the mechanisms that support pressure are apparently "reset" in hypertension and fight hard to keep the pressure up. As one mechanism is "knocked off" by a drug, the others fight even harder!

Even without knowing the specific cause of hypertension, we can select drugs that impair (but not obliterate) individual normal pressure-supporting systems. The effects of each drug will add to those of the other, and the sum can be normalized blood pressure without complete ruin of the kidneys, paralysis of the autonomic nervous system, or total relaxation of the blood vessels.

As a practical corollary to these principles, drugs are sequentially added in difficult cases, and the preceding drugs are continued. In many instances, dosage of the first or second drug can be reduced when the next one is added, but rarely is the first drug stopped completely. This leads to a scheme that resembles a staircase viewed from the side referred to as "stepped care." (Note that the staircase is solid; each succeeding step is built upon the preceding one.)

In some instances, individual drugs are more effective than one would have predicted from the early information about their mechanism of action. Further research has almost always indicated that the drugs possess multiple actions not originally understood. Thus, diuretics apparently affect peripheral arterioles as well as the kidneys, and hydralazine has an effect on the circulation of the kidneys as well as the peripheral arterioles. So some "single" agents are really intramolecular combinations.

The Steps of Stepped Care

Step One

1. *Diuretics* are ideal drugs for initiating therapy of hypertension. They will normalize pressure when used alone in almost half of all hypertensives.
2. The second advantage to diuretic therapy is the synergism it exerts with other modalities. As Guyton would have predicted, lowering the pressure, by any means other than renal, causes the kidneys to retain salt and water. Thus, other drugs alone, such as vasodilators, tend to lose effectiveness with time, because the kidneys start retaining fluid and cardiac output rises. Diuretics inhibit this compensatory renal effect.
3. There is some opinion favoring the use of β *blockers* alone as Step One therapy in young patients. Although they may be successful in a significant percentage of patients, β blocker side effects, when they occur, are not well-tolerated by young patients. Diuretics are better accepted

in that age group. Young people would rather have mild hyperuricemia than "mild" sedation or impotence! (For those patients who hate the effects of diuretics, β blockers are a good alternative.)

4. In the not-too-distant future, *converting enzyme inhibitors,* such as captopril, will be one alternative Step One therapy. These drugs have obvious logic supporting their use in patients with high plasma renin activities. Often, captopril and related drugs work surprisingly well as the only drug (monotherapy) for patients with normal renin levels.
5. The use of renin measurement to tailor initial therapy in hypertension is popular in some centers. Plasma renin activity (PRA) can detect those patients with "Low Renin Essential Hypertension," or those with "High Renin" (frequently from diseased kidneys or excessive adrenergic activity.) Patients with Low Renin Essential Hypertension may respond better to diuretics alone than will patients with high renin. Conversely, those with high renin may respond better to β blockers or converting-enzyme inhibitors alone. However, most patients respond to some degree to either drug regardless of the renin level. Renin measurement must be made under controlled conditions. (To uncover *low* renin levels, it is common to measure renin after two doses of furosemide to cause a diuresis, with the patient upright for 2 hr. Alternatively, the measurement can be made after a low-salt diet for 3 to 5 days.) The "renin profile" approach is probably more trouble than it is worth. It seems simpler to tailor therapy to side effects rather than to enzyme levels. Since diuretics, β blockers, and converting enzyme inhibitors are efficacious drugs, orchestration of their use should be determined by the patient's individual idiosyncrasies or intolerances. As renin and/or catecholamine measurements become more reliable and accessible, their levels may become increasingly useful in determining therapy.

Step Two

1. All of the traditional Step Two drugs act on the nervous systems—central and/or sympathetic.
2. *A β blocker* is an excellent choice for a second drug, to add to a diuretic in patients whose pressure does not normalize on diuretic alone. β Blockers attack the autonomic nervous system, a pressure-supporting mechanism not affected at all by diuretics. β Blockers prevent tachycardia that might result when a Step Three (vasodilator) drug is added, so the use of a β blocker at Step Two prepares the ground for possible use of a dilator later!
3. *Methyldopa* is commonly used today at Step Two. There are millions

of patients with normal pressure thanks to their use of a combination of diuretic and methyldopa. However, β blockers are rapidly eroding this market.

4. *Clonidine* is a reasonable selection at Step Two. It has no *a priori* contraindications. In other words, it is impossible to predict who will react badly to the drug. With propranolol, asthmatics and patients with heart block are clearly at increased risk of a bad drug reaction. With methyldopa, patients with liver or hematologic diseases are at risk. With clonidine, there are no clear contraindications. However, of all Step Two drugs, clonidine is the hardest to start, because the dry mouth and sedation that accompany its initial use are immediately obvious to the patient. With other Step Two drugs, side effects tend to take longer to develop.
5. Although considered a pariah by many, reserpine is an effective Step Two drug. At doses below 0.25 mg per day, it seldom causes depression. The combination of a diuretic plus reserpine is a smooth, gentle, effective regimen, achieving normal pressure in over 50% of all hypertensives.
6. The major deterrents to the use of either propranolol, methyldopa, clonidine or reserpine in a patient with no gross cardiac disease are the CNS side effects (sedation, depression, altered sleep or dream patterns). It is probably best to try one after another until the best compromise is reached. In this approach, the Step Two drugs are used one at a time. If one is unsuccessful, it is replaced by another, but the diuretic is continued.
7. *A converting-enzyme inhibitor* like captopril is the *most logical* Step Two drug. Angiotensin-converting enzyme (ACE) inhibitors block the major mechanism the body employs to antagonize diuretics (i.e., the renin–angiotensin system). Captopril is the obvious choice for patients with a high plasma renin to begin with. It could also be an ideal Step Two drug for patients who start out with normal or low renin, but whose renin system is triggered by the use of diuretics.
8. *Prazosin* is reasonable to try at Step Two. It also makes sense at Step Three, in combination with a diuretic plus a β blocker. Remember to watch out for that First-Dose Effect on postural hypotension and to build the dose up slowly from 1 mg. Doses as high as 30 mg per day can be used once the first dose has been successfully tolerated.

Step Three

1. A *vasodilator* is the logical drug to add to the regimen of a patient who has not achieved normal pressure despite the use of a diuretic and a

Step Two drug. The current favorite is *hydralazine*. It has the advantage of acting quickly and reversing quickly, so that dosage can be adjusted over short intervals. Hydralazine has the second (even more important) advantage of dilating renal arteries, so that renal blood flow is maintained even when pressure drops. This can be a significant factor in treating patients with impaired renal function from long-standing hypertension. When used in the presence of a β blocker and diuretic, hydralazine can be very effective at doses well below those where lupus syndrome is likely. Furthermore, the other major side effects of hydralazine—tachycardia, pounding headache, and flushing—are prevented by the β blocker.

2. *Prazosin* is a logical and useful choice for Step Three, especially when β blockers are already in use. β Blockers can cause vasoconstriction in those vessels where there are two kinds of opposing innervation: vasodilator β adrenergic and vasoconstrictor α adrenergic. The β blocker leaves α-constrictor activity unopposed. Prazosin can block α activity, so the net effect of both blockers is more effective. This combination would be very useful in patients with both coronary and peripheral arterial disease. The β blocker would lower cardiac output and reduce the need for coronary flow. Prazosin would help keep the leg vessels open!
3. *Captopril* is another logical Step Three drug. Its vasodilating activity is most evident in the presence of significant renin activity, and elevated renin activity is more likely in patients with severe hypertension than in milder cases.

Step Four

1. Patients who are not normalized when treated with a combination of diuretic, autonomic blocker, and vasodilator are considered "refractory" or "resistant." It is this group in which new drugs are tried and where more potent agents become useful. However, it is sometimes effective to add a fourth drug of moderate potency but with a mechanism of action different from the previous three.
2. *Guanethidine* is the traditional drug for treatment of patients resistant to a combination of diuretic, Step Two drug, and vasodilator. When guanethidine is invoked, previous drugs may need to be reduced in dosage. However, a diuretic is almost always needed, and a loop diuretic may also have to be started. Remember that the dominant adjunct to guanethidine usage is posture. Effects of this drug are very dependent on posture, and pressure can rise dramatically when the patient lies down. The most bothersome side effects of guanethidine are marks of autonomic imbalance: diarrhea and sexual dysfunction.

3. *Minoxidil* is a relatively new Step Four vasodilator drug. One would probably use it in place of hydralazine. Unlike hydralazine, this vasodilator does not open up the renal circulation, so dramatic sodium retention can follow a drop in pressure caused by minoxidil. This may require herculean doses of furosemide to overcome. More disconcerting to some patients than sodium retention is the widespread hair growth when minoxidil is used. It is conceivable that low doses of minoxidil will some day be used at Step Three in place of hydralazine, especially in patients who cannot tolerate the latter. There is little experience with this now.
4. *Captopril* (Capoten) is often useful for Step Four.
5. *Prazosin* may fine-tune a patient already receiving a diuretic, a β blocker, and a vasodilator. Beware of postural hypotension!
6. *Clonidine* is another drug that can be added at Step Four to a patient already receiving diuretic, β blocker and vasodilator. (It would *not* make sense to add it to a regimen that already included methyldopa.)

Other Drug Combinations

Diuretic Combinations

Addition of a potassium-sparing diuretic to a thiazide or loop diuretic is a logical and effective way to correct or prevent hypokalemia. Several combinations are available in single-tablet form. Probably the most widely used drug combinations contain hydrochlorothiazide plus spironolactone or triamterene (Aldactazide and Dyazide, respectively.) Moduretic is a new combination of thiazide and amiloride. There is some evidence that the combination of potassium-sparing drug with thiazide exerts a slightly better hypotensive effect as well as protecting against low K^+ levels.

In patients resistant to the effects of the powerful loop diuretics, better diuresis can be obtained often by adding a thiazide. One useful combination is furosemide plus metolazone. Although the thiazide is weaker than the loop diuretic, it acts at a different site in the nephron, preventing reabsorption downstream of the sodium blocked at the loop.

Other Combinations

SerApEs is a combination of reserpine (Serpasil®), hydralazine (Apresoline®), and hydrochlorothiazide (Esidrix®). It is a combination to be wary of, because the reserpine (whose presence in the tablet is not evident in the name) may produce depression. Several other tablets that contain reserpine are marketed under names that fail to announce that fact clearly. These include Enduronyl, Metatensin, Moderil, Rauzide, Sandril, Renese-R, Hydropres, Diupres, and Regroton. This is not deliberate obfuscation on the part of the marketing divisions of the companies. They simply want "catchy" names. However, it does present a threat to patients whose clinicians fail to examine closely the need or contraindications for reserpine and the contents of samples or promotional materials they may receive. On the other hand, these combinations offer significant convenience compared to multiple tablets.

There are many other combination tablets that contain a diuretic and a Step Two drug, such as aldomet or a β blocker. In general, one should prescribe these fixed-dose combination tablets when and if the patient has been titrated to those drugs and doses in a step-wise fashion.

Drug Resistance

There are two kinds of resistant patients: those whose disease is difficult to treat from the start and those whose hypertension responds to initial therapy, but who relapse during therapy. This section addresses itself only to the second kind, those who could be called "secondary failures." There are five common causes for "escape" from good hypertension control:

1. Failure to take the prescribed medicine ("noncompliance")
2. Fluid retention caused either by the lower pressure at the glomeruli of the kidneys after drug treatment or by worsening of renal disease
3. Renal artery stenosis resulting either from progression of atherosclerosis in the renal vessels or from narrowing of the renal vessels as the pressure is lowered
4. Treatment with nonsteroidal antiinflammatory drugs
5. Excessive alcohol ingestion

Noncompliance

The study of patient failure to take drugs is a science in itself. Noncompliance is far and away the chief cause of treatment failure. Certain features of hypertension and its treatment contribute to the high incidence of noncompliance. They include:

1. Hypertension is an asymptomatic condition. Patients have no internal goad to take drugs.
2. The benefits of taking medication are delayed, not immediate. Living longer is actually just dying later. Most people hate to think about their own death, acting as if immortal.
3. The medications invariably cause side effects. Unlike benefits, side effects of drugs are immediate and evident. Even low-dosage diuretics

cause many patients to feel weak. Impotence has even been attributed to diuretics alone (dubbed "penile syncope").

4. Medications invariably cost money, but the financial benefits of a longer life are not included in most people's budget calculations.
5. Medication routines can be complicated, with multiple types of drugs given at various times of the day. What seems so simple to the physician is a perplexing potpourri of pills to the patient.
6. Many patients feel that a good *response* to medication is tantamount to a *cure* of their hypertension. The fact that hypertension is usually INCURABLE, a lifelong affliction requiring life-long medication, is not palatable to most patients. Thus, when their pressures return to normal, they stop their drugs.
7. Many patients falsely attribute common symptoms to their hypertension, such as headache, anxiety, or flushed face. Therefore, when those unrelated symptoms abate, they stop their medication. All of these assumptions and conclusions are flawed. The symptoms are usually unrelated to pressure, and even if they were, their cessation would not justify discontinuation of therapy.

The best approaches to achieving compliance are to

1. Educate the patient *and* the patient's *family* about the disease. Emphasize the lack of symptoms, chronic nature, delayed dire effects, and the benefits of successful pressure reduction.
2. Equip all patients with a pressure cuff, so that they can participate actively in their own care. In addition, this device informs the practitioner about the levels of pressure the patient experiences during daily life.
3. Simplify the medication regimen. Most drugs can be given once or twice per day with good results. Diuretics can be given in the morning and almost all other drugs morning and evening. Drugs with a sedative side effect should be tried at bedtime alone, or the dose should be split with most of it given at night.
4. Question the patient about side effects, drug costs, and other concerns. Many people stifle their concerns from a sense of stoicism or because they feel that the practitioner should not be bothered with details. If the practitioner probes and can alleviate the problem, everyone will be happier and the treatment will be more successful. Office appointments should be kept promptly and made as pleasant, brief, and informative as possible.
5. Periodically *try to reduce drug doses*. Up to a fourth of treated patients do well with less or fewer drugs than their current regimen. This

should be considered every year or two. Less drug means fewer side effects.

Fluid Retention

Fluid retention that follows pressure reduction is to be expected, if Guyton is correct. Most patients do not suffer this if their diuretic is effective. Unfortunately, what causes diuresis at a high pressure may not at a lower pressure. Patients may also relax their salt restriction with time, so adequate diuresis at the start may not be adequate later in therapy. One way to detect this problem is by frequent checks of the patient's *weight*.

Treat fluid retention by two approaches:

1. Advise patient to reduce *salt intake*
2. Increase the *dose* or *potency of the diuretic*

Renal Artery Stenosis

Patients with an initially favorable response to therapy who become resistant to their standard drug regimen may be experiencing renin release from an ischemic kidney. Either the renal arteries have become plaqued and plugged, or the lower pressure has allowed occlusion by structural changes that were unimportant when the hypertension ballooned out the vessel.

One clue to this problem is a rise in serum creatinine or BUN. The rise that tips off the existence of renal artery stenosis is one that occurs later in therapy. (In many instances, there is a transient rise of BUN at the start of treatment in patients with bad kidneys. The BUN may rise, then fall over several weeks or months.) Measurement of plasma renin activity (PRA) can also be useful in deciphering this phenomenon. For example, propranolol should *lower* PRA. If a patient on propranolol (as well as other drugs) develops a *high* PRA, one should be suspicious of renal artery stenosis.

The real danger of this complication is the possibility that the kidney(s) will be badly compromised or infarcted by an over-zealous use of hypotensive drugs. It is better to search for a possible stenosis (listen for bruit, do a rapid-sequence IVP, or even an arteriogram) than to overcome it with brute pharmacologic force.

Nonsteroidal Antiinflammatory Drugs (NSAID's)

The pressure-lowering efficacy of many drugs depends in part on their ability to release prostaglandins. Such drugs include diuretics, vasodilators, and converting-enzyme inhibitors. It may also be true of some autonomic inhibitors.

NSAIDs all share the ability to inhibit prostaglandin release. If a hypertensive patient under good control is then given indomethacin (Indocin), ibuprofen (Motrin), phenylbutazone (Butazolidin), aspirin, or a similar agent, the blood pressure may rise.

The best way to overcome this problem is to raise the dose of antihypertensive drug, especially the diuretic, until the antiinflammatory agent can be discontinued. There is some evidence that one or more newer NSAIDs will be so selective that they will not affect antihypertensive drug action. That remains to be seen.

Alcohol Intake

Alcohol intake can confuse the picture in hypertensives. If your patient starts drinking more, he/she may escape from antihypertensive control. More than three drinks per day can elevate blood pressure. Furthermore, if the patient abstains from alcohol for a few hours before visiting the practitioner, pressure may soar as a manifestation of withdrawal!

Drug Selection

Confronted with a patient with elevated blood pressure who fails to respond to salt-restriction or other nondrug regimens, the medical practitioner is also confronted with a huge array of potential drug regimens from which to choose. The Stepped Care approach leaves a lot of latitude. Not only are there three main classes of drugs, each with several subclasses, but each group contains a myriad of minor molecular variations on each classical theme. Unfortunately, there is no simple guide through this garden of pharmacologic delights. The next chapter (Chapter 21) describes some special cases that lead to fairly *specific drug exclusions*. However, the majority of hypertensives do not have such conditions as renal failure, diabetes, or heart block, and do not assist in the choice of drugs by forcing the exclusion of some agents on medical grounds.

One way to select among the plethora of pharmaceutical products is to search the patient's history for clues that would *predict side effects*. Some examples are

1. If the patient has any evidence of bronchospasm or seasonal allergy, these conditions may be aggravated by nonspecific β blockers (instead consider clonidine, methyldopa or captopril at Step Two).
2. If the patient has any tendency to depression or sexual dysfunction, these tendencies may be converted to unpleasant side effects by drugs that affect the central nervous system (consider captopril at Step Two).

3. If the patient has a tendency to postural dizziness, that tendency may become significant postural hypotension with loop diuretics or prazosin (consider a β blocker or captopril at Step One).
4. If the patient has glucose intolerance or an elevated level of BUN or creatinine, he/she may suffer hyperkalemia more readily than normal patients when taking potassium-sparing diuretics or captopril (consider low doses of loop diuretics or a β blocker at Step One).
5. If the patient has hyperlipidemia, this condition might be aggravated by diuretics (consider β blockers or captopril at Step One).
6. If the patient has ever had pancreatitis, it might reappear with thiazide diuretics (consider captopril at Step One).

These and other similar scenarios constitute what are called the "relative contraindications" to use of certain drugs. Only by exclusion do they result in the selection of specific drugs for specific patients.

Finding reasons to exclude some drugs is a rather negative approach to the construction of a pharmacologic regimen. Are there *positive criteria* that can be *used?*

There have been some attempts to "type" hypertensive patients in ways that might dictate drug selection. Parameters such as plasma renin activity, pulse rate, cardiac output, and plasma volume have been measured. They have revealed at least two subtypes of hypertension: Low Renin Essential Hypertension, and Hyperdynamic–Hyperadrenergic Hypertension. Logic favors the use of diuretics at Step One in the former and β blockers in the latter. However, both groups of patients respond significantly to both classes of drugs, so the use of the "endocrine profile" or cardiac output determinations have not become very popular in general practice.

The most recent approach to selection of specific drugs is again based on side effects, but this time beneficial ones:

1. If the recent clinical trials with β blockers are substantiated and show that these drugs reduce mortality in patients with fresh myocardial infarction, consideration of β blockers will become almost mandatory in hypertensive patients with *recent* infarctions. It would also seem logical to use those drugs in patients at high risk for their *first* myocardial infarction, i.e., those with significant "risk factors" such as hyperlipidemia, strong family history, or glucose intolerance.
2. There is recent evidence that β blockers have therapeutic benefits in people with intolerable degrees of anxiety. In those patients, the "side effect" of mild sedation can be used to achieve therapeutic gain.
3. Drugs that lower serum uric acid as well as blood pressure are known. If a nontoxic member of this class becomes available, it will be useful to administer to patients with gout.

4. Patients with angina or migrane may obtain relief from these conditions (as well as from their hypertension) by use of β-blocker therapy.

The "two birds with one stone" approach is a method of drug selection that has a more positive ring than the avoidance of unpleasant side effects.

In summary, the Stepped Care approach to selection of antihypertensive drugs is a convenient, effective basis for treatment. Individualization of regimens within the framework, or deviations from it, are most logically based on avoidance of harmful or unpleasant side effects, and capitalization on beneficial side effects in selected patients.

21 Special Cases: Hypertension in Children, the Elderly, Pregnant Women, Preoperative Cases, and Patients with Other Diseases

Hypertension in Children

Introduction

The upper limits of normal blood pressure in children are now well known. This was not always so. For years, adult standards were applied to children. They are too high. Fig. 1 shows the current norms. Note that 120/75 becomes the average pressure only at age 14. At 6 or younger 100/60 is average and 120/80 must be considered hypertensive!

Obtaining accurate pressure measurements in children is frequently difficult.

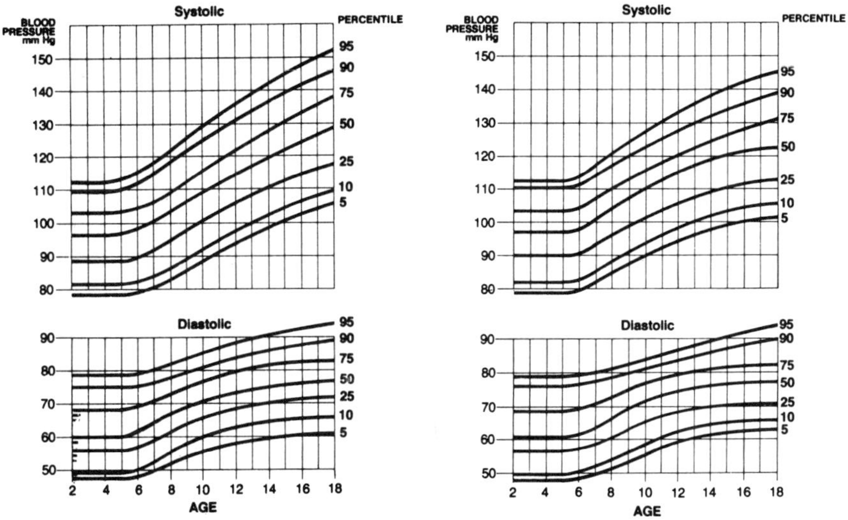

Fig. 1. Blood pressure norms (right arm, seated) of boys (left panels) and girls (right panels).

1. If Korotkoff sounds are not obtainable, one can use the palpated pulse, a Doppler flow probe, or a second cuff on the forearm to detect systolic pressure. (See details in Chapter 12.)
2. If Korotkoff sounds are audible, use phase IV (muffling) for diastole. There is often *no* phase V (sounds are heard down to 0).

Children tend to ''track'' within their peer group. Children with higher-than-average pressures at one age are likely to have higher-than-average pressures at older ages. A child's ''rank'' among his peers can be evident as early as the first few *months* of life! Therefore, pay special attention to children with *relatively* high pressures. Measure them regularly.

Etiology

Before puberty, the dominant causes of hypertension are *renal* diseases (up to 80%). The mechanisms by which these diseases cause hypertension are discussed in Chapter 4. The following are renal diseases that may cause hypertension in children.

1. Acute glomerulonephritis
2. Acute pyelonephritis
3. Nephrotic syndrome
4. Obstruction
5. Trauma

6. Congenital defects, such as polycystic disease
7. Renal arterial disease
8. Chronic renal failure
9. Lupus erythematosus
10. Hemolytic-uremic syndrome

It is always important to rule out *coarctation of the aorta*.

Adrenal cortical diseases, such as adrenogenital syndrome, other forms of congenital adrenal hyperplasia (CAH), and Cushing's syndrome can cause pediatric hypertension.

Rare *tumors*, such as neuroblastoma, pheochromocytoma, Wilms' tumor, or a renin-producing tumor can cause hypertension by virtue of the chemical pressors they release.

Increased intracranial pressure and *lead poisoning* can cause elevated arterial blood pressure in children.

Obesity is very commonly associated with essential hypertension in children. About half of those without other identifiable causes are obese.

Large stature (advanced development) leads to pressures more appropriate to the bone age than the chronologic age. Correct your normal range for the child's *size*, not age.

Genetic predisposition exerts a powerful influence in childhood hypertension. About half of the children with essential hypertension have a first-degree relative with hypertension.

Clinical Features

Symptoms of both the underlying disease (e.g., symptoms of renal disease) and the hypertension (e.g., headache) are much more common in affected children than in hypertensive adults.

The physical examination reveals eyeground changes (arteriolar spasm and A-V nicking) and cardiac findings (gallop rhythm, ventricular hypertrophy, heart failure). Remember to take the pressure in arms *and* legs and listen for the murmur of coarctation.

Urinalysis is *the* crucial laboratory exam.

An IVP should be performed (with rapid-sequence films) in all children with significant hypertension.

There is a tendency for hypertensive children to have higher levels of other cardiovascular risk factors (e.g., lipids and uric acid). Check these!

Therapy

Assuming that surgically correctable causes have been ruled out, the pressure level at which to treat with drugs and the level to strive for are *not clear*.

There are no long-term prospective studies in children to guide us. (Few investigators will outlive their pediatric subjects!) A reasonable approach is to attempt normalization by nondrug means and then to use mild drugs.

Advise the family to reduce its salt intake, using a "no-salt-added" diet. This is a safe and effective treatment.

Reduce the weight of obese children. This has several valuable fringe benefits.

Avoid nasal vasoconstrictors or other agents that elevate pressure pharmacologically.

When drugs are needed, consider β blockers and thiazides.

1. A β blocker alone, a diuretic alone, or a diuretic plus a β blocker will manage most cases.
2. Captopril shows great promise for children with severe renal disease.
3. In cases with proven adrenal dysfunction, suppress the pituitary–adrenal axis with corticoids to reduce secretion of abnormal steroids. Use spironolactone to block the effects of mineralocorticoids at their receptors if inoperable tumors are present.

In cases without demonstrable renal or adrenal disease, when conservative measures and drugs from steps one and two fail to drop the pressure below levels known to be life shortening in adults (140/90), consider adding vasodilators or ACE inhibitors such as captopril. It seems safe to assume that pressures that shorten the lives of adults will shorten the lives of children and that drugs will prove to do more good than harm over 50 years as they do over 10 years. The unfathomable question is what to do for children with pressures between 100/60 and 140/90.

Hypertension in the Elderly

Introduction

Hypertension is extremely prevalent in older populations; 30% of whites and 50% of blacks over 60 have elevated pressure.

Usually the *systolic* component dominates. Noncompliant atherosclerotic capacitance vessels, like the aorta, cannot accept the cardiac output gracefully. However, the majority of elderly hypertensives also have diastolic pressures somewhat higher than normal.

Atherosclerosis is both a cause and an effect of hypertension in this group. In young patients, atherosclerotic changes in the kidneys may or may not perpetuate hypertension. In the elderly, atherosclerosis of all vessels contributes to the pressure elevation.

The vascular damage caused by hypertension is more often fatal in the elderly than in the young or middle-aged. (In fact, *everything* is more lethal in older people.) Most of our ancestors died of coronaries, strokes, or cancer. Most people who die of the first two have hypertension! The risk of coronaries and stroke is increased threefold by a systolic pressure of 195, and the risk of congestive heart failure is increased sixfold.

Obesity is the most common identifiable contributing cause of hypertension in the elderly. Old age dampens activity before it dampens the appetite.

Occlusion of the renal arteries from atherosclerotic plaques is a cause of elevated pressure that becomes very significant in older patients, including those with preexisting hypertension from other causes. However, treatment by surgical repair is more risky in the elderly. (These are the patients where balloon dilatation of the artery may be most useful.)

Therapy

The recent, extensive HDFP study showed clearly that normalizing diastolic pressure in the elderly prolongs life. There was even a difference between the group whose diastolic pressure fell to 86 mm and those whose pressure fell to 81! The latter lived longer. Table I summarizes some of that data. This study justifies attempts to lower blood pressure all the way to 80 (diastolic) in everyone, regardless of age, race, or sex.

The guiding principle of therapy in the elderly is to *avoid postural hypotension.*

1. Most elderly patients have a low blood volume to begin with. About 25% will show a significant (20 mm) postural fall in pressure *before* therapy.
2. Elderly people often have weak baroreceptor reflexes. They get very little cardiac response to sudden changes in posture.
3. Be careful of causing excessive volume contraction by diuretics. Use them in low doses (e.g., 25–50 mg of hydrochlorothiazide per day).
4. Try to avoid using guanethidine and prazosin in the elderly. They have more postural side effects than other drugs.
5. Exercise special care with diabetics who may have autonomic dysfunction because of diabetic neuropathy. They may suffer particularly severe postural hypotension.
6. Beware of intercurrent events that can precipitously lower pressure, such as a hot, sweaty summer, a fever, a coronary occlusion, or a stroke. Adjust medications and replenish salt as needed in those instances.

TABLE I

Some Data from the Hypertension Detection and Follow-Up Program (HDFP), Showing Benefits of Strict Blood Pressure Control, Especially over Age 50

	Results of routine care			*Results of "stepped care"*			
	Blood pressure			*Blood pressure*			
Age	*Start*	*End*	*Deaths (%)*	*Start*	*End*	*Deaths (%)*	*Change in mortality with treatment (%)*
30–49	101	91	3.5	101	86	3.3	−6
50–59	101	88	8.3	101	84	6.2	−25
60–69	101	86	15.2	101	81	12.7	−16

7. If patients show postural hypotension with very little medication, consider the possibility that they have "pseudohypertension," i.e., *normal* intraarterial pressure but such *stiff pipes* that the *cuff pressure* must be extra-high to occlude the brachial artery.

Try salt restriction and weight reduction as initial modalities before going to drugs in treating the elderly.

Use gentle drugs at low doses.

1. A useful generalization is that elderly patients overrespond to drugs. (It is certainly true of their response to narcotics.) It may relate to their decreased volume of distribution or rate of excretion.
2. For a diuretic, use a thiazide and not furosemide. Use *half* the usual dose or less (e.g., 25 mg of hydrochlorthiazide once a day).
3. For Step Two, a β blocker has at least two possible advantages: it can lower systolic pressure without a disproportionate drop in diastolic pressure, because it reduces cardiac output, and it helps relieve any angina present.
4. Two other Step Two drugs useful in the elderly are clonidine and methyldopa. These drugs cause little postural hypotension, because they leave autonomic reflexes intact.

Current recommendations are to treat all diastolic hypertension in all patients, regardless of age. In patients with only systolic hypertension, treat if the systolic pressure is over 160; be content with lowering it to 140 to 160 and watch carefully for signs that low diastolic pressures are threatening vital organs.

Hypertension in Pregnancy

The clinician's worries are twofold in pregnant patients with hypertension: development of eclampsia if the pressure is untreated and feto-placental ischemia if it is overtreated.

The risk of *hypertension* itself is *not* so great that treatment is urgent at diastolic pressures under 110, *if* these pressures are achieved slowly. (A sudden burst to 110 can be lethal.) In other words, women with essential hypertension need *not* be treated vigorously simply because they become pregnant.

Watch for the ominous signs of imminent eclampsia:

1. Rapid pressure rise
2. Proteinuria
3. Abrupt weight gain or edema
4. Hyperreflexia
5. Falling urine output
6. Visual or cerebral symptoms
7. Pulmonary edema

Treat pregnant hypertensives with very high pressures with drugs affecting the autonomic nervous system or the vessels (not volume depletors). There is some evidence that diuretics reduce perfusion of the fetoplacental unit. Other data disagree and affirm their safety. Err on the conservative side. (Note that this is a deviation from the usual steps of stepped care.)

1. Use methyldopa, hydralazine, and/or a β blocker initially.
2. *Bed rest* is a very good mode of therapy, with emphasis on lying on the side. This position consistently lowers blood pressure in pregnant women.
3. Termination of pregnancy is always to be considered, especially if the fetus is sufficiently mature. In eclampsia, delivery results in dramatic cure of the disease, although seizures can occur up to three days later.
4. *Magnesium sulfate* is the best prophylaxis against *convulsions*. Although an old remedy, parenteral magnesium provides the best seizure prevention with the least depression of the fetus. The standard dose is 0.5 gm im, repeated every 2 hours, with neurological monitoring to avoid excessive CNS depression.

Anesthesia and Surgery in Hypertensives

When drugs that affected autonomic function became common in hypertensive treatment, anesthesiologists began to notice unusual responses in their patients. For example, reserpine causes hypersensitivity to catecholamines and propranolol blunts the cardiac response to everything. The initial reaction was to recommend that all drugs be stopped before surgery. That advice resulted in increased vascular accidents from hypertensive crises. As anesthesiologists learned to compensate for the drugs, their advice changed.

In brief, current wisdom is that the *treated* hypertensive is a better anesthetic risk than the *un*treated hypertensive. Pressure is more labile in untreated hypertensives, and surgery presents a rapidly changing series of perturbations to the cardiovascular system. Treatment reduces lability.

Discontinuing some drugs can lead to "rebound" effects. Angina or infarction have been seen after stopping propranolol and hypertensive crises after stopping clonidine. This emphasizes the value of *continued therapy*.

β Blockers may protect against arrhythmia during surgery, as well as contribute to control of blood pressure. They have now gained special favor, instead of being pariahs as they were before.

In summary, *control the pressure preoperatively* and *continue drugs* up to surgery whenever possible.

In anesthesia and surgery in hypertensive patients, be aware of the following:

1. Volume depletion can be dangerous in patients on diuretics. When these patients are anesthetized, vasodilation can drop the bottom out of their pressure support. Hemorrhage also obviously threatens the "dry" patient.
2. Postural lability of pressure is a problem in patients on guanethidine, prazosin, and those with contracted blood volume. As the head is lowered the pressure rises and vice versa.
3. The hypokalemia of those on thiazides may accentuate the effects of some muscle relaxants such as succinylcholine.
4. Postoperative hypertensive bursts are especially common after some types of surgery (e.g., procedures using heart–lung machines). These should be treated with short-lived parenteral agents such as hydralazine or nitroprusside while the patient is in the recovery room.

It is wise to resume hypertensive medications soon after surgery, using parenteral forms of the drugs if the patient is N.P.O. for a day or longer. Injectable hydralazine and methyldopa are available. Injectable propranolol must be given *very* carefully!

Treating Hypertension in Diabetics

It is even more important to lower pressure in diabetics than in nondiabetics. Hypertension dramatically escalates their risk of diabetic vascular complications, such as retinopathy and nephropathy.

Thiazide and loop diuretics will aggravate hyperglycemia in diabetics, increasing the need for insulin or oral hypoglycemic drugs. In general, this is a small problem relative to other aspects of diabetic management.

Potassium-sparing diuretics are life-threatening in diabetics, because two of their endocrine defenses against hy*per*kalemia are impaired (low insulin and hyporeninemic hypoaldosteronism), and they may also have impaired renal function. Insulin, aldosterone, and the kidneys all contribute to serum potassium regulation. Remember that insulin plus glucose is a good way to "drive" potassium into cells. (That combination can be used therapeutically to lower serum K^+). Thus, *deficient* insulin represents a weakened buffer to high K^+. It is a good idea to avoid potassium-sparing diuretics in all diabetics, e.g., spironolactone, triamterene, amiloride, and the combinations Aldactazide, Dyazide, and Moduretic.

Nonselective β blockers, like propranolol, by masking the symptoms of hypoglycemia (insulin reaction) and by blunting the metabolic buffer effected by epinephrine, make the "brittle" diabetic more subject to hypoglycemic shock. Such β blockers may also aggravate peripheral vascular disease, common in diabetics. Thus, it is a good idea to use β_1-selective β blockers in diabetics [e.g., metoprolol (Lopressor) and atenolol (Tenormin)].

Thiazides together with methyldopa, clonidine or prazosin are good combinations of drugs in diabetics. There is also a rationale for using low-dose loop diuretics once or twice per day in resistant diabetics. They yield more diuresis with less effect on blood sugar. ACE inhibitors such as captopril may be used in diabetics. They have no metabolic effects on glucose or insulin. However, ACE inhibitors reduce aldosterone secretion. Therefore, drugs like captopril may aggravate the tendency to high potassium levels in diabetes.

Treating Hypertension in Patients with Advanced Renal Disease

Pressure in patients with renal failure is either "volume dependent," or "volume independent." The former type of patient responds well to loss of fluid (by dialysis or diuresis). The volume *in*dependent patients do not respond to drying out. They usually have high renin levels caused by ischemic kidneys (that are more effective at their endocrine than their excretory functions).

Volume-dependent patients who can still respond to diuretics should receive them. These patients will almost always require loop diuretics. Loop diuretics work high enough in the nephron to increase urine flow, even when glomerular filtration is impaired. They also increase renal blood flow.

Thiazides alone do not work well in patients with renal disease. As a rule of thumb, switch to loop diuretics when the serum creatinine reaches 2 mg/dl.

Volume *in*dependent patients need ACE inhibitors, vasodilators, and/or β blockers in addition to loop diuretics. Captopril has been a miracle drug for some renal patients with hypertension. If high renin production cannot be treated by surgical repair or removal of the kidneys, no other drug can approach the usefulness of ACE inhibitors in blocking the renin system. These patients may ultimately require nephrectomy. (Nephrectomy sometimes occurs spontaneously, the ischemic kidney infarcts as pressure is lowered with drugs.)

The favorite pure vasodilator in renal failure is hydralazine, because it increases renal blood flow. Captopril may also work if the vasoconstriction is mediated by angiotensin. Remember, however, that excessive reduction of pressure can induce renal failure. Even a sick kidney requires perfusion.

Remember, patients with renal failure will *retain many drugs* (as well as creatinine, potassium, and urea). Therefore, they may get along well with normal doses at longer intervals or with reduced doses at the usual intervals. Fortunately, blood pressure can be monitored so that overdosage of antihypertensive drugs is readily detected.

It is essentially *forbidden to use potassium-sparing diuretics in renal failure!*

Other Diseases

Heart Disease

Although virtually all adults with hypertension have some left ventricular hypertrophy, that condition is not enough to affect the choice of drugs. (There is some evidence that vasodilators alone might not be as effective in reversing hypertrophy as drugs that slow the heart rate.) However, patients who have progressed to symptomatic coronary atherosclerosis or heart failure present some problems in antihypertensive care.

In the presence of coronary atherosclerosis with angina or evidence of infarction, be very wary of pure vasodilators known to increase the heart rate. If drugs such as hydralazine, minoxidil, or diazoxide are needed, buffer the pulse rate with a little β blocker, methyldopa, or even reserpine.

In the presence of frank or incipient congestive heart failure, β blockers may reduce the strength of contraction of the left ventricle to a dangerous degree. It is safer to lower the pressure by other means. Although there are many instances of successful treatment with β blockers in the presence of failure (because the drop in pressure did the heart more good than the lower inotropy did harm), this is a high risk drug choice. (If too much inotropy is lost by adding β blocker, it might be restored by injecting glucagon. Glucagon adds inotropy without using adrenergic receptors.)

When digitalis is given, patients become susceptible to ventricular tachyarrhythmias, and that tendency is aggravated by low serum K^+. Be careful to maintain the normal level of serum K^+ whenever digitalis is used. The use of diuretic combinations containing a potassium-sparing agent is a convenient way to do this.

Patients with variant angina (Prinzmetal type), who have worse pain at night than during the day and whose ST-T segments go down instead of up, often have more pain with β blockers. (Most angina patients have less pain with β blockers.) Apparently, some of the problem in variant angina is caused by coronary artery spasm, partly mediated by α-adrenergic or cholinergic receptors. When β blockers are given, the dilatory β receptors are blocked, and the constrictor receptors are unopposed. If angina gets worse with use of a β blocker, odds are it is variant angina. These patients should not be given β blockers for their hypertension. Prazosin makes much more sense. (They may also need a calcium-channel blocker such as nifedipine or a nitrate to dilate directly their coronary arteries.)

Atherosclerosis

Again, virtually all hypertensives have accelerated atherosclerosis compared to normotensives. But some aspects of therapy bear directly on the atherosclerosis itself.

All patients begun on diuretics should have their cholesterol checked before and a few months after initiating therapy. Some will experience marked increases in total and LDL cholesterol (the "bad" cholesterol is LDL, the "good" is HDL). If this response is seen, switch from a diuretic to a β blocker or to an ACE inhibitor as monotherapy.

Patients with severe peripheral vascular disease may do poorly on β blockers that are nonspecific. These blockers eliminate the β_2 (vasodilator) adrenergic responses that help to maintain peripheral circulation. If this happens, switch to a specific β blocker (such as metoprolol or atenolol), or switch to a non-β-blocker Step Two drug, such as prazosin.

Pulmonary Disease

Patients with all varieties of pulmonary disease tend to have some degree of bronchospasm, not just those with asthma.

Be very careful when treating hypertension with β blockers in any patient with pulmonary disease. These patients may depend on β_2 receptors to keep their bronchi open. Although the selective blockers are supposed to be better, they are only relatively selective, and at full dosage they block the bronchodilatory β_2 receptors as well as the cardiac β_1 receptors.

The better part of valor in treating pulmonary patients with hypertension is to treat with Step Two drugs other than β blockers. Consider methyldopa, clonidine, prazosin, or captopril.

Depression

Naturally, one should avoid treating depressed hypertensive patients with drugs known to aggravate depression (e.g., reserpine and centrally acting autonomic blockers such as methyldopa and β blockers). ACE inhibitors such as captopril are an excellent alternative at Step Two or Three. Hydralazine also has no effect on mood. Prazosin has very little effect on the brain.

Patients taking lithium excrete less of it when given diuretics. Therefore, reduce the dose of lithium by one-third to one-half when adding a diuretic. Whatever you do, monitor the serum lithium level until things stabilize.

Arthritis

Remember the antagonism between nonsteroidal antiinflammatory drugs and many antihypertensive drugs. The dose of the latter may have to be increased to overcome the former.

22 Hypertensive Crises

Introduction

The term ''Hypertensive Crisis'' is usually understood to mean ''Malignant Hypertension,'' a condition marked by an accelerated rise in pressure over hours or days (instead of years) and rapid pathology in the vessels, brain, eyes, and kidneys. However, a better definition should also include *any acutely dangerous condition* in which the *blood pressure contributes* to the problem and in which the *patient would improve quickly if the pressure were lowered*.

Using the broader definition, conditions such as congestive heart failure with only mildly elevated blood pressure would be included; so would uncontrollable arterial bleeding, or dissection of the aorta, even when the pressure itself was only slightly above normal.

Malignant Hypertension

Clinical Findings

Naturally, there is *high pressure,* almost always *over 120 diastolic,* frequently over 140.

The eyegrounds show *hemorrhages, exudates,* a ''wet'' shiny retina, and *papilledema.* (The patient may complain of altered vision.)

The characteristic central nervous system symptoms and signs include headache, nausea, confusion, somnolence or coma, and focal neurological deficits or seizures. This picture is called ''Hypertensive Encephalopathy.''

The real tip-off is deteriorating renal function, marked by rising BUN and creatinine levels and a *less-than-normal output of water and salt.* Falling urine output is the danger signal that may precede neurological findings or papilledema. The renal filler is ''plugged,'' there is no overflow valve for an expanded blood volume, and the increased pressure is not relieved by increasing urine output.

Frequently, there are signs of *heart failure* (as well as the hypertrophy caused by any underlying chronic hypertension).

Laboratory Findings

The urine contains *protein and red cells.*

The blood chemistry shows azotemia. Remember the BUN rises faster than the creatinine after any acute reduction in renal function.

Plasma renin activity is usually elevated, with secondary hyperaldosteronism.

Red blood cells may appear fragmented on smear (''microangiopathic hemolytic anemia''). This is thought to be caused by actual trauma to the cells as they are banged around under pressure through tight arterioles.

The electroencephalogram (EEG) shows focal abnormalities.

Previous History

The pressure level at which malignant hypertension develops depends on the ''premalignant'' pressure and the rate at which the acute rise occurs. Chronically hypertensive patients *resist* conversion to the malignant phase. Their cerebral vessels autoregulate to keep flow constant over a broad range of pressures, and their peripheral vessels are ''protected'' by preexisting hypertrophy.

By contrast, previously normal patients who experience sudden rises of pressure (e.g., eclampsia, treatment with MAO inhibitors plus tyramine-rich foods, pheochromocytoma "attacks," or sudden renal artery occlusions) suffer severe damage to vessels and target organs at relatively low pressures.

Today, a common cause of malignant hypertension is the sudden cessation of antihypertensive therapy in a patient with moderate-to-severe hypertension.

Pathology (see Chapter 11)

Malignant hypertension is characterized by fibrinoid necrosis of arterioles, progressing to necrotizing arteriolitis and necrotizing glomerulitis. (Note the common use of term "necrosis" in this sentence. This condition actually kills cells in the vessel wall.)

Thickening of the intima in renal vessels leads to an "onion-skin" appearance.

Pathogenesis

A vicious circle is established in which renal failure and renin secretion are *induced* by high pressure, with the renal abnormalities *contributing* to further pressure elevation. Furthermore, loss of the renal "safety valve" of pressure diuresis aggravates any underlying cause of hypertension.

Renin release establishes a new cause for hypertension. Renin release is probably the result of damage to the vessels in the glomeruli and spasm of the afferent arterioles.

Cerebral edema may set off a CNS drive to increased pressure, establishing a second vicious circle.

There may be increased secretion of vasopressin (ADH).

Some investigators feel that immune or inflammatory mechanisms may be involved in malignant hypertension.

Prognosis

Ninety percent of untreated patients with malignant hypertension are dead in 6 months if their eyegrounds show papilledema. With treatment, 80% live one year.

Early in the disease, death occurs from renal failure and stroke. With longer survival, deaths are more likely to result from heart failure.

Treatment

Reducing pressure by *any* means breaks the vicious cycles in malignant hypertension. The release of renin from bludgeoned JG cells stops when the excessive pressure drops. Even though a fall in pressure stimulates release of renin in normals, plasma renin levels usually fall with falling pressure in malignant hypertension.

Although renal function may deteriorate at first, it usually improves as pressure drops with successful therapy. Apparently, stopping the hammering on renal vessels allows them to dilate and serve the excretory function better. Inflammatory responses to this injury also abate if the pressure is lowered.

Malignant hypertension is a medical emergency that can be successfully treated by drugs that are readily available and reasonably well understood. This previously hopeless situation is now a manageable emergency. The mainstays of therapy are powerful vasodilators and diuretics.

1. The cornerstone of therapy in a situation where pressure monitoring is available is nitroprusside (Nipride®). To administer this agent, add one vial (50 mg) to a 500-cc bottle of 5% dextrose in water; cover the bottle with foil to keep out light that can accelerate deterioration of the nitroprusside and drip in the mixture iv at a rate designed to administer from 0.5 to 3.0 mcg per kg per min. (The bottle with one vial per 500 cc has 100 mcg per ml. One ml per min would deliver 1.4 mcg per kg to a 70-kg patient.) The rate of dripping must be determined by the desired dose and the size of the drops. Microdrop dispensers obviously require more drops. The average dose is 3 mcg per kg per min. Do not push past 10 mcg per kg per min. Monitor the patient closely, and adjust the drop rate as needed.
2. The second-best vasodilator drug for hypertensive emergencies is diazoxide (Hyperstat®). This must be administered in short, fast bolus injections intravenously. (It is in alkaline diluent and will burn if extravasated from the vein.) The dose first recommended was 200–300 mg. This dose overshot the desired effect in some patients, and caused excessive hypotension. Now, it is common to give smaller boluses of 60–100 mg, each one in a short burst, and to repeat after 5 to 10 min if the pressure does not drop adequately. It is not necessary to monitor the patient as closely after diazoxide as during nitroprusside.
3. If nitroprusside and diazoxide are out of stock or out of favor, intravenous hydralazine can be used.
4. There are a few published reports of the successful use of clonidine or captopril in hypertensive emergencies. Clonidine might cause sedation that might mimic the cerebral changes of hypertensive encephalopathy. Both of these agents will probably be useful in selected patients.
5. Finally some people like trimethaphan camsylate (Arfonad), a gang-

lion blocker that effectively lowers almost anyone's pressure. Like nitroprusside, it must be monitored closely.

6. No matter which vasodilator (or ganglion blocker) is used, *treatment must include a loop diuretic,* usually intravenous furosemide (Lasix), given in a dose of about 40 mg. This is an essential and integral part of therapy for malignant hypertension.
6. When careful monitoring of the patient is not possible (e.g., in a patient treated at home), one intramuscular dose of *reserpine* (1.0–2.0 mg) can be used. This often gives smooth pressure reduction without depression. It can take hours instead of minutes to do the job.
8. If catecholamine ingestion (or clonidine withdrawal or a pheochromocytoma) is part of the pathogenesis, use prazosin or phentolamine (Regitine) to block α-adrenergic receptors. In these crises, the "first dose" effect of prazosin can be a blessing.
9. Start your long-term therapy (such as a β blocker, plus hydralazine or captopril) *from the very beginning* of hospitalization. The acute treatment drugs cannot be used indefinitely and the less exotic agents become more effective after a few days of administration. It is hoped that the chronic therapy will hold the pressure down by the time the intravenous drugs are stopped.

Other Emergencies involving Elevated Blood Pressure

Dissecting Aortic Aneurysm

Whatever the pressure is when the aorta begins to shear, that pressure is too high. It is urgent to relieve the strain on the aorta and the shearing force of the blood.

β Blockers are the cornerstone of therapy. They will lower pressure and "soften" the cardiac impulse, and the volume and speed of left ventricular ejection will be reduced. All of these effects reduce the shearing force on the aorta.

Avoid agents, such as hydralazine or diazoxide, that increase the force of cardiac contraction.

It would be valuable to use a vasodilator that would allow rapid run-off of the cardiac output and spare the aorta. However, vasodilators that trigger tachycardia and *increase* cardiac output would be counterproductive. *Nitroprusside* is an ideal stop-gap agent. Converting-enzyme inhibitors such as captopril and prazosin are very helpful for long-term therapy.

Furosemide keeps the kidneys open despite decreased blood pressure, reduces intravascular volume, and further lowers cardiac output and arterial blood pressure. As in other hypertensive emergencies furosemide is very useful in aortic dissection.

Left Ventricular Failure

The patient in congestive heart failure has an imbalance between the capacity of the left ventricle to eject blood and the demands placed on the ventricle by venous return and the organs it must perfuse. One way to reduce demand is to reduce arterial pressure. (Congestive failure may also contribute to high arterial blood pressure because of increased sympathetic outflow.)

To lower arterial pressure without starving the perfused organs, use a vasodilator like nitroprusside, prazosin, captopril or hydralazine. These vasodilators reduce cardiac "afterload," the load against which the heart must pump during systole. This greatly reduces the energy requirement of the left ventricle and may restore the balance between the heart's capability and its responsibility.

The traditional approach to congestive failure—*diuresis*—is obviously a good idea for patients with greater arterial pressure than they need or can pump. This attack on "preload" has its limits. Below a certain level, central venous pressure can be suboptimal for cardiac output.

The *converting-enzyme inhibitors show great promise* for management of heart failure with or without hypertension. They dilate both arteries and veins, and often open up the renal circulation as well, promoting diuresis.

Whatever the vasodilator, it must be titrated against the reduced perfusion of vital organs that results when pressure falls too low.

Pheochromocytoma Exacerbation or Drug Reaction

In such cases (e.g., overdose of pressor agent or MAO inhibitor plus pressor amine):

1. Give *phentolamine* (Regitine) iv. Prazosin is a logical oral drug.
2. Follow these α blockers with β blockers. *Never use a β blocker first.*

23 Future Trends in Hypertension

Etiology

The two known contributors to hypertension are heredity and the environment. Recent work on the hereditary aspect has involved the following reasoning:

1. If genetic theory applies to hypertension, then the abnormal gene(s) of the hypertensive are present in every nucleated cell, and the abnormal gene product(s) may be expressed in several cell types. Perhaps an abnormality of only one cell type is sufficient to produce hypertension. (It might be an abnormal tubule cell in the kidney causing slight sodium retention.) Yet, there might be many cell types with a biochemically identical abnormality, even if it did *not* contribute to elevated pressure by its expression in those cells.
2. Some investigators have found an abnormality in the red cells of hypertensive patients and their not-yet-hypertensive relatives. The abnormality involves a sodium leak. Although apparently irrelevant to the red cell, this kind of abnormality expressed in a kidney cell could affect sodium excretion, in a vascular cell it could cause swelling and vasoconstriction, and in the brain it might trigger excessive discharges of the pressor type. Even if wrong, this idea reflects the best type of biochemical approach to the genetic contribution to hypertension.

With respect to the environment, almost all past effort was directed toward salt (i.e., sodium) and calories in the diet. Some newer ideas include the following:

1. Some investigators suspect that trace metals, like cadmium, might cause subtle damage to the kidneys and elevate the pressure. This might explain the association of hypertension with industrial civilizations.
2. It is a common finding that people with a high sodium intake also have a low potassium intake. The effects of high salt intake can be partially neutralized by high potassium fed at the same time. Potassium has a mysterious protective action, keeping pressure low despite high sodium. This may result from an effect of potassium on the kidneys. It is a subject of considerable interest and great therapeutic promise.
3. If salt is indeed the major environmental culprit, intake could be reduced by a cheap, tasty salt substitute. Nothing is available that really tastes like salt.
4. There is some evidence for a role for calcium in hypertension. A calcium ''leak'' in the kidneys, a calcium deficiency, or some other circumstance results in a slightly lower serum calcium in hypertensive patients compared to controls. The implications of this finding for the prevention or treatment of hypertension are many, but much more research is required.

Two organs that receive a lot of attention with respect to etiology are the arterioles and the brain:

1. There is a consensus that adults who have had elevated pressure for years will continue to have it, even if the initiating cause disappears. They are thought to have thickened vessels, especially involving the peripheral arterioles and the arteries in the kidneys. At such a stage, lowering the pressure with drugs does not result in a cure, because the thickened vessels never thin out and dilate again. There are glimmers of suggestions that some agents can inhibit synthesis of collagen and connective tissue and enable vessels to return to their pristine, dilated state. Most of the suggested agents are too toxic to consider, but it is a thought worth pursuing.
2. Because the brain is so obviously active in maintaining pressure and because so many drugs apparently act there, much research is focussed on understanding pressure regulation mechanisms in the central nervous system. Most promising is the elucidation of the neurotransmitters that might be active at the regulatory centers. Current favorites include the catecholamines such as dopamine, and GABA (γ-amino-

butyric acid). Each new transmitter is examined for its possible role, but there are no other hot leads. (Apparently, the endogenous opioids such as enkephalins are mere bit-players even though morphine invariably lowers blood pressure).

Perhaps the most popular type of research in hypertension is discovering *endogenous substances that affect blood pressure*.

1. As mentioned in the chapter on hyperaldosteronism, researchers are actively seeking new chemicals that stimulate aldosterone secretion. One such substance, excreted in the urine, apparently comes from the pituitary gland. Prolactin and insulin are also likely candidates. So is one form of MSH (melanocyte stimulating hormone).
2. New mineralocorticoids are proposed annually. 18-Hydroxydeoxycorticosterone (18-OH-DOC) was popular for a time. Now, 19-nor-deoxycorticosterone (19-nor-DOC) is a very promising candidate. These might explain forms of hypertension in which renin levels are low. The adrenal cortex remains a fertile ground for biochemical burrowing.
3. It is tempting to think of hypertension by analogy to hyperglycemia. If the analogy is appropriate, hypertension may be caused by a *deficiency* of *de*pressor substances, just as diabetes is caused by deficiency of insulin. If so, which depressor is deficient?
4. The products of arachidonic acid metabolism, including the prostaglandins, prostacyclins, and thromboxanes, have been thought responsible for everything from arthritis to "the Blahs." The most potent vasoconstrictor known is thromboxane; however, it is so labile and short-lived it cannot be bottled. It is logical to attribute hypertension to excess thromboxane or to deficient vasodilators. Unfortunately, no firm evidence to support that idea has been produced.
5. Because of the clearly deleterious effects of dietary salt, it has been proposed that hypertension is caused by deficient endogenous diuretics, leading to salt accumulation. This has led to searches for endogenous diuretics (also called "Third Factor," the third factor regulating sodium excretion in addition to glomerular filtration and aldosterone). Identification of these substances has so far eluded us. There is accumulating evidence for an endogenous equivalent of digitalis. Such a substance could affect blood pressure and renal sodium excretion by inhibiting membrane Na^+/K^+-ATPase. A diuretic peptide has recently been found in cardiac (atrial) tissue.
6. Finding new pressure-regulating functions for old substances is an active research topic. The role of catecholamines, especially nor-

epinephrine and dopamine, in the handling of sodium and potassium by the kidneys is being studied. Apparently, norepinephrine is a salt retainer and dopamine is a diuretic. They may act via changes in circulation within the kidney.

7. Vasopressin (antidiuretic hormone) is another well-known substance that may participate in development or maintenance of hypertension. We will not know its role for certain until a long-acting antagonist is available.
8. The most tantalizing clinical situation related to hypertension is eclampsia. Towering blood pressures drop to normal upon delivery of the fetus and placenta. If that condition is not caused by a circulating pressor substance, what is? So far, all attempts to prove the existence or nature of the chemical(s) causing eclampsia have failed.

New insights into receptor physiology suggest that hypertension, with its high set-point but normal regulatory loops, may be the result of *bad receptors*. Perhaps the hypertensive's pressure-sensors need more of a signal to respond. Perhaps the effectors respond too vigorously.

The physiologic event that seems most relevant to long-term blood pressure regulation (outside of renal sodium excretion) is autoregulation. The mechanism whereby arterioles constrict or dilate to adjust flow in response to tissue demand and arterial pressure is not understood. Oxygen, pH, potassium, adenosine, lactate, and other chemicals have been proposed. Understanding eludes us.

Diagnosis

Early diagnosis of the hypertensive "diathesis" (or "tendency") would enable early institution of preventive measures, such as salt restriction. The test of red cell leaks mentioned above is one approach. Another is the renal response to a salt load. Apparently, adult relatives of hypertensives excrete a load of salt slower than do controls. This suggests that Guyton is right and that a subtle defect of renal sodium handling is truly a part of the hypertensive state. There is also evidence that some people respond to a salt load with a greater hypertensive response than others do. Translation of these observations into a clinically useful test has not been achieved.

A simple screening test for each of the curable causes of hypertension would be valuable. One novel approach to hyperaldosteronism was the measurement of the electrical potential across the colonic epithelium. Since aldosterone activates sodium reabsorption there, it is logical that the potential difference be increased by the hormone. Thus, an electrode inserted rectally was devised. Sure enough, the potential was higher in the rectum of patients with higher aldosterone. For reasons that should have been anticipated by the investigators, this method never caught on.

Many patients live a normal lifespan with elevated pressures. Apparently, their vessels are resistant to its damaging effects. Others go to pieces with mild elevations. It would be valuable to have diagnostic tests that would detect the susceptibles. So far, only the well-known risk-factor measurements are available. (An earlier suggestion that patients with low renin levels were immune from vascular disease has not been confirmed.)

Treatment

The big news in therapy in the 1980's will be a series of converting-enzyme inhibitors. They will all probably be equally efficacious, differing only in their side effects. They should make a clear and lasting contribution to therapy.

The type of drug most needed (among the classical types) is a good, mild vasodilator with activity on the renal vessels (a safer equivalent of hydralazine). The best candidates so far are the "calcium channel blockers" (e.g., nifedipine). They paralyze smooth muscle at the cell membrane. They will almost surely play a role in hypertension management, although it is too soon to say exactly how.

It would be lovely to have a diuretic that did not either waste or conserve potassium, one that simply acted on sodium reabsorption. This would have to be an agent that worked on or beyond the aldosterone site, since the response to diuresis always includes some degree of hyperaldosteronism.

Another approach to diuresis would be to use an agent like spironolactone that is a competitive inhibitor of aldosterone. Using this type of drug leaves a safety valve: when the aldosterone level gets high enough, it overcomes the competitive block. A more potent, less toxic spironolactone would be useful.

It is likely that new drugs will be developed that can affect specific sites in the nervous system. If so, a targeted agent that could reset the autonomic centers regulating blood pressure, but not affect other brain functions, would be a useful drug. We can see glimmers of the effect such a drug could exert in the results now obtained from reserpine, clonidine, and methyldopa. More specific versions of these agents are needed.

Finally, to overcome noncompliance, we need a very long-acting form of a nontoxic drug, or something that we can add to table salt or the drinking water! At this time, noncompliance rather than lack of efficacy limits successful therapy.

Prevention

All efforts at prevention have involved attempts to modify salt and calorie ingestion. There is virtually nothing new in this area. It remains the most appealing of all approaches to the epidemic problem of hypertension. This is where our major need lies. Any ideas?

Answers to Practice Grid in Chapter 5

Clinical condition	*Blood volume*	*Aldo (in blood or urine)*	*Renin (in peripheral blood)*	*K^+ (blood)*	*K^+ (urine)*	*Na^+ (urine)*
Primary hyperaldosteronism	↑	↑	↓	↓	↑	↓
Dehydration	↓	↑	↑	—[a]	—[a]	↓
Licorice fetish	↑	↓	↓	↓	↑	↓
Cirrhosis with ascites	↓	↑	↑	—[a]	—[a]	↓
Renal tubular defect causing Na^+ retention	↑	↓	↓	↓	↑	↓

[a] Total urine flow is low, so there is not much loss of potassium.

Bibliography

General

Genest J, Koiw E, Kuchel O (eds.): *Hypertension*. New York, McGraw-Hill, 1977.

Kaplan NM: *Clinical Hypertension*. Baltimore, Williams & Wilkins, 1978.

McMahon, FG: Management of Essential Hypertension. Mt. Kisko, New York, Futura, 1978.

Chapter 1

Brody MJ, Haywood JR, Touw KB: Neural mechanisms in hypertension. *Ann Rev Physiol* 42:441–453, 1980.

Guyton AC: *Human Physiology and Mechanisms of Disease*, ed 3. Philadelphia, W.B. Saunders, 1982, pp 178–186.

Guyton AC: *Arterial Pressure and Hypertension*. Philadelphia, W.B. Saunders, 1980.

Guyton AC, Coleman TG, Cowley AW, Jr, Scheel KW, Manning RD, Jr, Norman RA, Jr: Arterial pressure regulation. Overriding dominance of the kidneys in long-term regulation and in hypertension. *Am J Med* 52:584–594, 1972.

Haddy FJ: 'Local control of vascular resistance as related to hypertension. *Arch Intern Med* 133:916–931, 1974.

Laragh JH, Sealey JE, Niarchos AP, Pickering TG: The vasoconstriction-volume spectrum in normotension and in the pathogenesis of hypertension. *Fed Proc* 41:2415–2423, 1982.

Page IH: The mosaic theory of arterial hypertension—Its interpretation. *Perspect Biol Med* 10:325–333, 1967.

Schmid PG, Abboud FM: Neurohumoral control of vascular resistance. *Arch Intern Med* 133:935–945, 1974.

Chapter 2

Bartter FC: Bartter's syndrome: A disorder of vascular reactivity. *Hypertension* 3(suppl I):I-69–I-73, 1981.

Davis JO, Freeman RH: Mechanisms regulating renin release. *Physiol Rev* 56:1–56, 1976.

Erdos EG: Conversion of angiotensin I to angiotensin II. *Am J Med* 60:749–759, 1976.

Kaplan NM: Renin profiles. The unfulfilled promises. *JAMA* 238:611–613, 1977.

Keeton TK, Campbell WB: The pharmacologic alteration of renin release. *Pharmacol Rev* 31:81–227, 1981.

Laragh JH, Letcher RL, Pickering TG: Renin profiling for diagnosis and treatment of hypertension. *JAMA* 241:151–156, 1979.

Page LB: Clinical value of plasma renin determinations in renovascular and primary hypertension. *Am Heart J* 91:665–672, 1976.

Peach MJ: Renin-angiotensin system: Biochemistry and mechanisms of action. *Physiol Rev* 57:313–370, 1977.

Perez GO, Lespier L, Jacobi J, Oster JR, Katz FH, Vaamonde CA, Fishman LM: Hyporeninemia and hypoaldosteronism in diabetes mellitus. *Arch Intern Med* 137:852–855, 1977.

Phelps KR, Lieberman RL, Oh MS, Carroll HJ: Pathophysiology of the syndrome of hyporeninemic hypoaldosteronism. *Metabolism* 29:186–199, 1980.

Reid IA, Morris BJ, Ganong WF: The renin-angiotensin system. *Ann Rev Physiol* 40:377–410, 1978.

Chapter 3

Langer SZ: Presynaptic regulation of the release of catecholamines. *Pharmacol Rev* 32:337–362, 1980.

Mayer SE: Neurohumoral transmission and the autonomic nervous system, in Gilman AG, Goodman JS, Gilman A (eds): *The Pharmacological Basis of Therapeutics*. New York, MacMillan, 1980, pp 56–90.

Mendlowitz M, Vlachak ND: The catecholamines in essential hypertension. *Am Heart J* 91:378–382, 1976.

Chapter 4

Atkinson AB, Brown JJ, Cumming AMM, Fraser R, Lever AF, Leckie BJ, Morton JJ, Robertson JIS, Davies DL: Captopril in the management of hypertension with renal artery stenosis: Its long-term effect as a predictor of surgical outcome. *Am J Cardiol* 49:1460–1466, 1982.

Chasis H, Baldwin DS: The kidney in essential hypertension. Victim or culprit. *Circulation* 34:921–924, 1966.

Ferris TF: The kidney and hypertension. *Arch Intern Med* 142:1889–1895, 1982.

Foster JH, Maxwell MH, Franklin SS, Bleifer KH, Trippel OH, Juliam OC, DeCamp PT, Varady PT: Renovascular occlusive disease. Results of operative treatment. *JAMA* 231:1042–1048, 1975.

Franklin SS, Young JD Jr, Maxwell MH, Foster JH, Palmer JM, Cerny J, Varady PD: Operative morbidity and mortality in renovascular disease. *JAMA* 231:1148–1153, 1975.

Grim CE, Luft FC, Weinberger MH, Grim CM: Sensitivity and specificity of screening tests for renal vascular hypertension. *Ann Intern Med* 91:617–622, 1979.

Hollenberg NK, Borucki LJ, Adams DF: The renal vasculature in early essential hypertension: Evidence for a pathogenetic role. *Medicine* 57:167–178, 1978.

Hunt JC, Sheps SG, Harrison EG Jr, Strong CG, Bernatz PE: Renal and renovascular hypertension. A reasoned approach to diagnosis and management. *Arch Intern Med* 133:988–999, 1974.

Lankford NS, Donohue JP, Grim CE, Weinberger MH: Results of surgical treatment of renovascular hypertension. *J Urol* 122:439–441, 1979.

Madias NE, Millan VG: PTRA in the treatment of renovascular hypertension. *Hosp Prac* August:105–116, 1981.

Onesti G, Kim KE, Greco JA, del Guercio ET, Fernandes M, Swartz C: Blood pressure regulation in end-stage renal disease and anephric man. *Circ Res* 36(suppl I):I-145–I-152, 1975.

Schwarten DE, Yune HY, Klatte EC, Grim CE, Weinberger MH: Clinical experience with percutaneous transluminal angioplasty (PTA) of stenotic renal arteries. *Radiology* 135:601–604, 1980.

Shapiro AP, McDonald RH Jr, Scheib E: Renal arterial stenosis and hypertension. II. Current criteria for surgery. *Am J Cardiol* 37:1065–1068, 1976.

Stanley JC, Fry WJ: Surgical treatment of renovascular hypertension. *Arch Surg* 112:1291–1297, 1977.

Starr DS, Lawrie GM, Morris GC Jr: Surgical treatment of renovascular hypertension. Long-term follow-up of 216 patients up to 20 years. *Arch Surg* 115:494–496, 1980.

Tegtmeyer CJ, Dyer R, Teates CD, Ayers CR, Carey RM, Wellons HA Jr, Stanton LW: Percutaneous transluminal dilatation of the renal arteries. *Radiology* 135:589–599, 1980.

Tobian L Jr: Hypertension and the kidney. *Arch Intern Med* 133:959–967, 1974.

Youngberg SP, Sheps SG, Strong CG: Fibromuscular disease of the renal arteries. *Med Clin North Am* 61:623–641, 1977.

Chapter 5

Brown RD, Wisgerhof M, Carpenter PC, Brown G, Jiang N-S, Kao P, Hegstad R: Adrenal sensitivity to angiotensin II and undiscovered aldosterone stimulating factors in hypertension. *J Steroid Biochem* 11:1043–1050, 1979.

Coghlan JP, Blair-West JR, Denton DA, Fei DT, Fernley RT, Hardy KJ, McDougall JH, Puy R, Robinson PM, Scoggins BA, Wright RD: Control of aldosterone secretion. *J Endocr* 81:55P–67P, 1979.

Edmonds CJ, Richards P: Measurement of rectal electrical potential difference as an instant screening-test for hyperaldosteronism. *Lancet* September:624–628, 1970.

Ferriss JB, Beevers DG, Brown JJ, Davies DL, Fraser R, Lever AF, Mason P, Neville AM, Robertson JIS: Clinical, bochemical and pathological features of low-renin (''primary'') hyperaldosteronism. *Am Heart J* 95:375–388, 1978.

Ganguly A, Pratt JH, Yune HY, Grim CE, Weinberger MH: Detection of adrenal tumors by computerized tomographic scan in endocrine hypertension. *Arch Intern Med* 139:589–590, 1979.

Herf SM, Teates DC, Tegtmeyer CJ, Vaughan ED Jr, Ayers CR, Carey RM: Identification and differentiation of surgically correctable hypertension due to primary aldosteronism. *Am J Med* 67:397–402, 1979.

Streeten DHP, Tomycz N, Anderson GH Jr: Reliability of screening methods for the diagnosis of primary aldosteronism. *Am J Med* 67:403–413, 1979.

Weinberger MH, Grim CE, Hollifield JW, Kem DC, Ganguly A, Kramer NJ, Yune HY, Wellman H, Donohue JP: Primary aldosteronism. Diagnosis, localization, and treatment. *Ann Intern Med* 90:386–395, 1979.

Chapter 6

Bravo EL, Tarazi RC, Gifford RW, Stewart BH: Circulating and urinary catecholamines in pheochromocytoma. Diagnostic and pathophysiologic implications. *N Engl J Med* 301:682–686, 1979.

Ganguly A, Henry DP, Yune HY, Pratt JH, Grim CE, Donohue JP, Weinberger MH: Diagnosis and localization of pheochromocytoma. Detection by measurement of urinary norepinephrine excretion during sleep, plasma norepinephrine concentration and computerized axial tomography (CT-scan). *Am J Med* 67:21–26, 1979.

Lawrence AM: Glucagon provocative test for pheochromocytoma. *Ann Intern Med* 66:1091–1096, 1967.

Manger WM, Gifford RW, Jr: *Pheochromocytoma*. New York, Springer-Verlag, 1977.

Chapter 7

Maron BJ, Humphries JO, Rowe RD, Mellits ED: Prognosis of surgically corrected coarctation of the aorta. A 20-year postoperative appraisal. *Circulation* 47:119–126, 1973.

Ribeiro AB, Krakoff LR: Angiotensin blockade in coarctation of the aorta. *N Engl J Med* 295:148–150, 1976.

Chapter 8

Fisch IR, Frank J: Oral contraceptives and blood pressure. *JAMA* 237:2499–2503, 1977.

Klatsky AL, Friedman GD, Siegelaub AB, Gerard MJ: Alcohol consumption and blood Pressure. Kaiser-permanente multiphasic health examination data. *N Engl J Med* 296:1194–1200, 1977.

Lipsett MB, Combs JW Jr, Catt K, Seigel DG: Problems in contraception. *Ann Intern Med* 74:251–263, 1971.

Weinberger MH: Oral contraceptives and hypertension. *Hosp Prac* May:65–75, 1975.

Chapter 9

Ferris TF: Managing toxemia in pregnancy. *Resident and Staff Physician* March:49–57, 1978.

Gilstrap LC, III, Cunningham FG, Whalley PJ: Management of pregnancy-induced hypertension in the nulliparous patient remote from term. *Semin Perinatol* 2:73–81, 1978.

Pritchard JA: Management of Severe Preeclampsia and eclampsia. *Semin Perinatol* 2:83–97, 1978.

Wilson M, Morganti AA, Zervoudakis I, Letcher RL, Romney BM, Von Oeyon P, Papera S, Sealey JE, Laragh JH: Blood pressure, the renin-aldosterone system and sex steroids throughout normal pregnancy. *Am J Med* 68:97–104, 1980.

Chapter 10

Arkwright PD, Beilin LJ, Rouse I, Armstrong BK, Vandogeń R: Effects of alcohol use and other aspects of lifestyle on blood pressure levels and prevalence of hypertension in a working population. *Circulation* 66:60–66, 1982.

Dahl LK: Salt intake and salt need. *N Engl J Med* 258:1152–1208, 1958.

Freestone S, Ramsay LE: Effect of coffee and cigarette smoking on the blood pressure of untreated and diuretic-treated hypertensive patients. *Am J Med* 73:348–353, 1982.

Freis ED: Salt, volume and the prevention of hypertension. *Circulation* 53:589–595, 1976.

Frohlich ED, Tarazi RC, Dustan HP: Hyperdynamic β-adrenergic circulatory state. *Arch Intern Med* 123:1–7, 1969.

Ganguly A, Weinberger MH: Low renin hypertension: A current review of definitions and controversies. *Am Heart J* 98:642–652, 1979.

Gibson GS, Gibbons A: Hypertension among blacks. An annotated bibliography. *Hypertension* 4:I-1–I-52, 1982.

Grim CE, Luft FC, Miller JZ, Rose RJ, Christian JC, Weinberger MH: An approach to the evaluation of genetic influences on factors that regulate arterial blood pressure in man. *Hypertension* 2(suppl I):I-34–I-42, 1980.

Kannel WB, Wolf PA, McGee DL, Dawber TR, McNamara P, Castelli WP: Systolic blood pressure, arterial rigidity, and risk of stroke. The Framington study. *JAMA* 245:1225–1229, 1981.

McCarron DA: Low serum concentrations of ionized calcium in patients with hypertension. *N Engl J Med* 307:226–228, 1982.

Messerli FH, Ventura HO, Reisin E, Dreslinski GR, Dunn FG, MacPhee AA, Frohlich ED: Borderline hypertension and obesity: Two prehypertensive states with elevated cardiac output. *Circulation* 66:55–60, 1982.

Page LB: Epidemiologic evidence on the etiology of human hypertension and its possible prevention. *Am Heart J* 91:527–534, 1976.

Pickering G: Hypertension. Definitions, natural histories and consequences. *Am J Med* 52:570–583, 1972.

Stamler J, Stamler R, Rhomberg P, Dyer A, Berkson DM, Reedus W, Wannamaker J: Multivariate analysis of the relationship of six variables to blood pressure: Findings from Chicago community surveys, 1965–1971. *J Chron Dis* 28:499–525, 1975.

Stamler J, Rhomberg P, Schoenberger JA, Shekelle RB, Dyer A, Shekelle S, Stamler R, Wannamaker J: Multivariate analysis of the relationship of seven variables to blood pressure: Findings of the Chicago Heart Association detection project in industry, 1967–1972.

Chapter 11

Lynch RP, Edwards JE: Pathology of systemic hypertension including background and complications. In Hurst JW (ed), *The Heart, Arteries and Veins,* ed3. New York, McGraw-Hill, 1974, pp 1179–1189.

Pickering G: Hypertension. Definitions, natural histories and consequences. *Am J Med* 52:570–583, 1972.

Rabinowitz M: Overview on pathogenesis of cardiac hypertrophy. *Circ Res* 34,35(suppl II):II-3–II-11, 1974.

Chapter 12

Caldwell JR: Practical approach to hypertension. 1. Diagnostic evaluation. *Postgrad Med* 65:66–77, 1979.

Cohn JN, Limas CJ, Guiha NH: Hypertension and the heart. *Arch Intern Med* 133:969–979, 1974.

Franceschi M, Tancredi O, Smirne S, Mercinelli A, Canal N: Cognitive processes in hypertension. *Hypertension* 4:226–229, 1982.

Gifford RW: Evaluation of the hypertensive patient. *Chest* 64:336–339, 1973.

Grim CE, Weinberger MH, Higgins JT, Kramer NJ: Diagnosis of secondary forms of hypertension. *JAMA* 237:1331–1335, 1977.

Hypertension Detection and Follow-Up Program Cooperative Group: Blood pressure studies in 14 communities. A two-stage screen for hypertension. *JAMA* 237:2385–2391, 1977.

Katz FH: Practical evaluation of hypertension. *Resident and Staff Physician* May:82–86, 1975.

Sandok BA, Whisnant JP: Hypertension and the brain. *Arch Intern Med* 133:947–954, 1974.

Shapiro AP, Miller RE, King HE, Ginchereau EH, Fitzgibbon K: Behavioral consequences of mild hypertension. *Hypertension* 4:355–360, 1982.

The Joint National Committee on Detection, Evaluation, and Treatment of High Blood Pressure: The 1980 report of the Joint National Committee on Detection, Evaluation, and Treatment of High Blood Pressure. *Arch Intern Med* 140:1280–1285, 1980.

Wilkins RW, Hollander W, Chobanian AV: *Evaluation of Hypertensive Patients*. CIBA Pharmaceutical Company, Summit, New Jersey, 1972.

Chapter 13

Benson H: Systemic hypertension and the relaxation response. *N Engl J Med* 296:1152–1156, 1977.

Freis ED: Should mild hypertension be treated? *N Engl J Med* 307:306–309, 1982.

Hunt JC: Management and treatment of essential hypertension. in Genest J, Koiw E, Kuchel O (eds), *Hypertension*. New York, McGraw-Hill, 1977, pp 1068–1085.

Hypertension Detection and Follow-up Program Cooperative Group: Five-year findings of the Hypertension Detection and Follow-up Program. I. Reduction in mortality of persons with high blood pressure, including mild hypertension. *JAMA* 242:2562–2571, 1979.

Hypertension Detection and Follow-up Program Cooperative Group: The effect of treatment on mortality in ''mild'' hypertension. Results of the hypertension detection and follow-up program. *N Engl J Med* 307:975–980, 1982.

Marsh AC, Klippstein RN, Kaplan SD: *The Sodium Content of Your Food*. United States Department of Agriculture, Home and Garden Bulletin Number 233, 1980.

Miller NE, Dworkin BR: Effects of learning on visceral functions—Biofeedback. *N Engl J Med* 296:1274–1278, 1977.

Multiple Risk Factor Intervention Trial Research Group: Multiple risk factor intervention trial. Risk factor changes and mortality results. *JAMA* 248:1465–1477, 1982.

Pickering G: Hypertension. Definitions, natural histories and consequences. *Am J Med* 52:570–583, 1972.

Pooling Project Cooperative Group: Relationship of blood pressure, serum cholesterol, smoking habit, relative weight and ECG abnormalities to incidence of major coronary events. *J Chronic Dis* 31:201–306, 1978.

Reisin E, Abel R, Modan M, Silverberg DS, Eliahou HE, Modan B: Effect of weight loss without salt restriction on the reduction of blood pressure in overweight hypertensive patients. *N Engl J Med* 298:1–6, 1978.

Shapiro AP, Schwartz GE, Ferguson DCE, Redmond DP, Weiss SM: Behavioral methods in the treatment of hypertension. A review of their clinical status. *Ann Intern Med* 86:626–636, 1977.

Stamler J: Epidemiology of coronary heart disease. *Med Clin North Am* 57:5–46, 1973.

Veterans Administration Cooperative Study Group on Antihypertensive Agents: Effects of treatment on morbidity in hypertension. II. Results in patients with diastolic blood pressure averaging 90 through 114 mm Hg. *JAMA* 213:1143–1149, 1970.

Chapter 14

Allen JM, Hind CRK, McMichael HB: Synergistic action of metolazone with loop diuretics. *Br Med J* 282:1873, 1981.
Ames RP, Hill P: Elevation of serum lipid levels during diuretic therapy of hypertension. *Am J Med* 61:748–757, 1976.
Beyer KH: The basis for modern diuretic therapy. *Clin Ther* 1:425–443, 1978.
de Carvalho JGR, Dunn FG, Lohmoller G, Frohlich ED: Hemodynamic correlates of prolonged thiazide therapy: Comparison of responders and nonresponders. *Clin Pharmacol Ther* 22:875–880, 1977.
Dirks JH: Mechanisms of action and clinical uses of diuretics. *Hosp Prac* September:99–110, 1979.
Finnerty FA, Jr, Maxwell MH, Lunn J, Moser M: Long-term effects of furosemide and hydrochlorothiazide in patients with essential hypertension. *Angiology* 28:125–133, 1977.
Freis ED: Hemodynamic changes during acute and chronic administration of thiazide diuretics. In Sambhi MP (ed): *Systemic Effects of Antihypertensive Agents,* New York, Symposia Specialists, 1976.
Ram CVS, Reichgott MJ: Treatment of loop-diuretic resistant edema by the addition of metolazone. *Curr Ther Res* 22:686–691, 1977.
Royer RJ: Progress in the treatment of hypertension: A multicentre study of indapamide in 442 patients. *Curr Med Res Opin* 5:151–156, 1977.
Winer BM, Lubbe WF, Colton T: Antihypertensive actions of diuretics: Comparative study of an aldosterone antagonist and a thiazide, alone and together. *JAMA* 204:775–779, 1968.

Chapter 15

Bia MJ, DeFronzo RA: Extrarenal potassium homeostasis. *Am J Physiol* 240:F257–F268, 1981.
Cheng JT, Sapir DG, Turin MD, Walker WG: A comparison of potassium bicarbonate and potassium chloride in the repair of potassium deficiency. *Johns Hopkins Med J* 133:299–311, 1973.
Dyckner T, Wester PO: Ventricular extrasystoles and intracellular electrolytes before and after potassium and magnesium infusions in patients on diuretic treatment. *Am Heart J* 97:12–18, 1979.
Holland OB, Nixon JV, Kuhnert L: Diuretic-induced ventricular ectopic activity. *Am J Med* 70:762–768, 1981.
Hulting J: In-hospital ventricular fibrillation and its relation to serum potassium. *Acta Med Scand Suppl* 647:109–116, 1980.
MacLeod SM: The rational use of potassium supplements. *Postgrad Med* 57:123–128, 1975.
Morgan T, Myers J: Potassium maintenance. Potassium supplements or potassium sparing agents. *Acta Med Scand Suppl* 647:117–123, 1980.
Nordrehaug JE: Malignant arrhythmias in relation to serum potassium values in patients with an acute myocardial infarction. *Acta Med Scand Suppl* 647:101–107, 1980.

Schwartz AB, Swartz CD: Dosage of potassium chloride elixir to correct thiazide-induced hypokalemia. *JAMA* 230:702–704, 1974.

Solomon RJ, Cole AG: Importance of potassium in patients with acute myocardial infarction. *Acta Med Scand* 647:87–99, 1980.

Tan SY, Shapiro R, Franco R, Stockard H, Mulrow PJ: Indomethacin-induced prostaglandin inhibition with hyperkalemia. A reversible cause of hyporeninemic hypoaldosteronism. *Ann Intern Med* 90:783–785, 1979.

Whang R, Aikawa JK: Magnesium deficiency and refractoriness to potassium repletion. *J Chron Dis* 30:65, 1977.

Chapter 16

Anderson RJ, Hart GR, Crumpler CP, Reed WG, Matthews C: Oral clonidine loading in hypertensive urgencies. *JAMA* 246:848–850, 1981.

Awan NA, Mason DT: Oral vasodilator therapy with prazosin in severe congestive heart failure. *Am Heart J* 101:695–700, 1981.

Barnes PJ, Wilson NM, Vickers H: Prazosin, an alpha$_1$-adrenoreceptor antagonist, partially inhibits exercise-induced asthma. *J Allergy Clin Immunol* 68:411–415, 1981.

Bjorkqvist SE: Clonidine in alcohol withdrawal. *Acta Psychia Scand* 52:256–263, 1975.

Carstairs KC, Breckenridge A, Dollery CT, Worlledge SM: Incidence of a positive direct coombs test in patients on α-methyldopa. *Lancet* July:133–152, 1966.

Cobaugh DS: Prazosin treatment of ergotamine-induced peripheral ischemia. *JAMA* 244:1360, 1980.

Colucci WS, Wynne J, Holman BL, Braunwald E: Long-term therapy of heart failure with prazosin: A randomized double blind trial. *Am J Cardiol* 45:337–344, 1980.

Garbus S, Weber MA, Proest RT, Brewer DD, Hubbell FA: The abrupt discontinuation of antihypertensive treatment. *J Clin Pharmacol* August–September:476–486, 1979.

Gold MS, *et al:* Clonidine in acute opiate withdrawal. *N Engl J Med* 302:1421–1422, 1980.

Graham RM, Pettinger WA: Prazosin. *N Engl J Med* 300:232–236, 1979.

Horwitz D, Pettinger WA, Orvis H, Thomas TE, Sjoerdsma A: Effects of methyldopa in fifty hypertensive patients. *Clin Pharmacol Ther* 8:224–234, 1967.

Jain AK, Ryan JR, Vargas R, McMahon FG: Efficacy and acceptability of different dosage schedules of clonidine. *Clin Pharmacol Ther* 21:382–387, 1977.

Lilja M, Jounela AJ, Juustila H, Mattila MJ: Interaction of clonidine and β-blockers. *Acta Med Scand* 207:173–176, 1980.

Lowenstein J: Diagnosis and treatment. Drugs five years later. Clonidine. *Ann Intern Med* 92:74–77, 1980.

Maddrey WC, Boitnott JK: Hepatitis induced by isoniazid and methyldopa. *Hosp Prac* April:119–125, 1975.

Mroczek WJ, Leibel BA, Finnerty FA, Jr: Comparison of clonidine and methyldopa in hypertensive patients receiving a duiretic. *Am J Cardiol* 29:712–717, 1972.

Reid JL, Dargie JH, Davies DS, Wing LMH, Hamilton CA, Dollery CT: Clonidine withdrawal in hypertension. Changes in blood-pressure and plasma and urinary noradrenaline. *Lancet* June:1171–1174, 1977.

Thananopavarn C, Golub MS, Eggena P, Barrett JD, Sambhi MP: Clonidine, a centrally acting sympathetic inhibitor, as monotherapy for mild to moderate hypertension. *Am J Cardiol* 49:153–158, 1982.

Waldo R: Prazosin relieves Raynaud's vasospasm. *JAMA* 241:1037, 1979.

Chapter 17

Formgren H: The effect of metoprolol and practolol on lung function and blood pressure in hypertensive asthmatics. *Br J Clin Pharmac* 3:1007–1014, 1976.

Frishman W: Clinical pharmacology of the new beta-adrenergic blocking drugs. Part 1. Pharmacodynamic and pharmacokinetic properties. *Am Heart J* 97:663–670, 1979.

Frishman W, Silverman R: Clinical pharmacology of the new beta-adrenergic blocking drugs. Part 2. Physiologic and metabolic effects. *Am Heart J* 97:797–807, 1979.

Frishman W, Silverman R: Clinical pharmacology of the new beta-adrenergic blocking drugs. Part 3. Comparative clinical experience and new therapeutic applications. *Am Heart J* 97:119–131, 1979.

Frishman W, Silverman R, Strom J, Elkayam U, Sonnenblick E: Clinical pharmacology of the new beta-adrenergic blocking drugs. Part 4. Adverse effects. Choosing a β-adrenoreceptor blocker. *Am Heart J* 97:256–262, 1979.

Frishman WH: β-Adrenoceptor antagonists: New drugs and new indications. *N Engl J Med* 305:500–506, 1981.

Frishman WH: Beta-adrenergic blockade in clinical practice. *Hosp Prac* September:57–68, 1982.

Hjalmarson A, Herlitz J, Malek I, Ryden L, Vedin A, Waldenstrom A, Wedel H, Elmfeldt D, Holmberg S, Nybert G, Swedberg K, Waagstein F, Waldenstrom J, Wilhelmsen L, Wilhelmsson C: Effect on mortality of metoprolol in acute myocardial infarction. *Lancet* October:823–827, 1981.

James IM, Griffith DNW, Pearson RM, Newbury P: Effect of oxprenolol on stage-fright in musicians. *Lancet* November:952–954, 1977.

Lager I, Smith U, Blohme G: Effect of cardioselective and nonselective β-blockade on the hypoglycemia response in insulin-dependent diabetics. *Lancet* March:458–461, 1979.

Man In'T Veld AJ, Schalekamp MADH: How intrinsic sympathomimetic activity modulates the haemodynamic responses to β-adrenoceptor antagonists. A clue to the nature of their antihypertensive mechanism. *Br J Clin Pharmac* 13:245S–257S, 1982.

Molinoff PB, Aarons RD, Nies AS, Gerber JG, Wolfe BB, Goens MB: Effects of pindolol and propranolol on β-adrenergic receptors on human lymphocytes. *Br J Clin Pharmac* 13:365S, 1982.

Textor SC, Fouad FM, Bravo EL, Tarazi RC, Vidt DG, Gifford RW, Jr: Redistribution of cardiac output to the kidneys during oral nadolol administration. *N Engl J Med* 307:601–605, 1982.

Tsukiyama H, Otsuka K, Higuma K: Effects of β-adrenoceptor antagonists on central haemodynamics in essential hypertension. *Br J Clin Pharmac* 13:269S–278S, 1982.

Veterans Administration Cooperative Study Group on Antihypertensive Agents: Comparison of propranolol and hydrochlorothiazide for the initial treatment of hypertension. II. Results of long-term therapy. *JAMA* 248:2004–2011, 1982.

Chapter 18

Boston Collaborative Drug Surveillance Program: Reserpine and breast cancer. *Lancet* September:669–671, 1974.

Curb JD, Hardy RJ, Labarthe DR, Borhani NO, Taylor JO: Reserpine and breast cancer in the hypertension detection and follow-up program. *Hypertension* 4:307–311, 1982.

Kedia K, Markland C: The effect of pharmacological agents on ejaculation. *J Urol* 114:569–573, 1975.

Mitchell JR, Cavanaugh JH, Arias L, Oates JA: Guanethidine and related agents. III. Antagonism by drugs which inhibit the monorepinephrine pump in man. *J Clin Invest* 49:1596–1604, 1970.

Prichard BNC, Johnston AW, Hill ID, Rosenheim ML: Bethanidine, guanethidine, and methyldopa in treatment of hypertension: A within-patient comparison. *Brit Med J* 1:135–144, 1968.

Veteans Adminstration Cooperative Study Group on Antihypertensive Agents: Propranolol in the treatment of essential hypertension. *JAMA* 237:2303–2310, 1977.

Weinshilboum RM: Series on pharmacology in practice. 8. Antihypertensive drugs that alter adrenergic function. *Mayo Clin Proc* 55:390–402, 1980.

Chapter 19

Aldigier, J-C, Plouin P-F, Guyene TT, Thibonnier M, Corvol P, Menard J: Comparison of the hormonal and renal effects of captopril in severe essential and renovascular hypertension. *Am J Cardiol* 49:1447–1452, 1982.

Atkinson AB, Brown JJ, Fraser R, Leckie B, Lever AF, Morton JJ, Robertson JIS: Captopril in hypertension with renal artery stenosis and in intractable hypertension; acute and chronic changes in circulating concentrations of renin, angiotensins I and II and aldosterone, and in body composition. *Clin Sci* 57:139s–143s, 1979.

Captopril Collaborative Study Group: Does captopril cause renal damage in hypertensive patients? *Lancet* May:988–990, 1982.

Case DB, Atlas SA, Laragh JH, Sealey JE, Sullivan PA, McKinstry DN: Clinical experience with blockade of the renin-angiotensin-aldosterone system by an oral converting-enzyme inhibitor (SQ 14,225, captopril) in hypertensive patients. *Prog Cardiovasc Dis* 21:195–206, 1978.

Case DB, Atlas SA, Marion RM, Laragh JH: Long-term efficacy of captopril in renovascular and essential hypertension. *Am J Cardiol* 49:1440–1446, 1982.

Cushman DW, Cheung HS, Sabo EF, Ondetti MA: Design of new antihypertensive drugs: Potent and specific inhibitors of angiotensin-converting enzyme. *Prog Cardiovasc Dis* 21:176–182, 1978.

Gavras H, Waeber B, Gavras I, Biollaz J, Brunner HR, Davies RO: Antihypertensive effect of the new oral angiotensin converting enzyme inhibitor "MK-421." *Lancet* Setpember:543–546, 1981.

Gottlieb TB, Katz FH, Chidsey CA, III: Combined therapy with vasodilator drugs and beta-adrenergic blockage in hypertension. *Circulation* XLV:571–582, 1972.

Grim CE, Luft FC, Grim CM, Klotman PE, Van Huysse JW, Weinberger MH: Rapid blood pressure control with minoxidil. Acute and chronic effects on blood pressure, sodium excretion, and the renin-aldosterone system. *Arch Intern Med* 139:529–533, 1979.

Hollenberg NK: Renal response to angiotensin-converting enzyme inhibition. *Am J Cardiol* 49:1425–1429, 1982.

Linas SL, Nies AS: Minoxidil. *Ann Intern Med* 94:61–65, 1981.

Miller WE, Gifford RW Jr, Humphrey DC, Vidt DG: Management of severe hypertension with intravenous injections of diazoxide. *Am J Cardiol* 24:870–875, 1969.

Moser M: Diazoxide—An effective vasodilator in accelerated hypertension. *Am Heart J* 87:791–795, 1974.

Pettinger WA: Minoxidil and the treatment of severe hypertension. *N Engl J Med* 303:922–926, 1980.

Streeten DHP, Anderson GH, Dalakos TG: Angiotensin blockade: Its clinical significance. *Am J Med* 60:817–824, 1976.

Vidt DG, Bravo EL, Fouad FM: Captopril. *N Engl J Med* 306:214–218, 1982.

Wenting GJ, De Bruyn JHB, Man In't Veld AJ, Woittiez AJJ, Derkx FHM, Schalekamp MADH: Hemodynamic effects of captopril in essential hypertension, renovascular hypertension and cardiac failure: Correlations with short- and long-term effects on plasma renin. *Am J Cardiol* 49:1453–1459, 1982.

Chapter 20

Bulpitt CJ, Dollery CT: Side effects of hypotensive agents evaluated by a self-administered questionnaire. *Br Med J* 3:485–490, 1973.

Caldwell JR: Practical approach to hypertension. 2. Treatment. *Postgrad Med* 65:81–92, 1979.

Durao V, Martins Prata MM, Pires Goncalves LMP: Modification of anti-hypertensive effect of β-adrenoceptor-blocking agents by inhibition of endogenous prostaglandin synthesis. *Lancet* November:1005–1007, 1977.

Dustan HP, Page IH, Tarazi RC, Frohlich ED: Arterial pressure responses to discontinuing antihypertensive drugs. *Circulation* 37:370–379, 1968.

Editorial: Trials and tribulations of a symptom-free hypertensive physician receiving the best of care. *Lancet* August:291–292, 1977.

Finnerty FA, Jr: Step-down therapy in hypertension. Importance in long-term management. *JAMA* 246:2593–2596, 1981.

Gifford RW Jr: Managing hypertension. *Postgrad Med* 61:153–163, 1977.

Patak RV, Mookerjee BK, Bentzel CJ, Hysert PE, Babej M, Lee JB: Antagonism of the effects of furosemide by indomethacin in normal and hypertensive man. *Prostaglandins* 10:649–659, 1975.

Stokes GS, Oates HF, MacCarthy EP: Antihypertensive therapy: New pharmacological approaches. *Am Heart J* 100:741–751, 1980.

Swartz SL, Williams GH: Angiotensin-converting enzyme inhibition and prostaglandins. *Am J Cardiol* 49:1405–1409, 1982.

Veterans Administration Cooperative Study Group on Antihypertensive Agents: Comparison of propranolol and hydrochlorothiazide for the initial treatment of hypertension. II. Results of long-term therapy. *JAMA* 248:2004–2011, 1982.

Veterans Administration Cooperative Study Group on Antihypertensive Agents: Comparison of propranolol and hydrochlorothiazide for the initial treatment of hypertension. I. Results of short-term titration with emphasis on racial differences in response. *JAMA* 248:1996–2003, 1982.

Chapter 21

Finnerty FA, Jr: Hypertension in the elderly. Special considerations in treatment. *Postgrad Med* 65:199–125, 1979.

Jesse MJ: Essential hypertension in children. *Hosp Prac* November:81–88, 1982.

Katz RL: Hazardous effects of drugs in hypertensive patients scheduled for elective surgery. *Cardiovasc Med* November:1185–1205, 1978.

Kilcoyne MM: The developing phase of primary hypertension. I. Identification of the problem. *Mod Concepts Cardiovasc Dis* XLIX:19–24, 1980.

Kilcoyne MM: The developing phase of primary hypertension. II. Treatment. *Mod Concepts Cardiovasc Dis* XLIX:25–30, 1980.

Kirkendall WM, Hammond JJ: Hypertension in the elderly. *Arch Intern Med* 140:1155–1161, 1980.

Knowler WC, Bennett PH, Ballintine EJ: Increased incidence of retinopathy in diabetics with elevated blood pressure: A six year follow-up study in Pima Indians. *N Engl J Med* 302:645–650, 1980.

Lager I, Smith U, Blohme G: Effect of cardioselective and nonselective β-blockade on the hypoglycaemic response in insulin-dependent diabetics. *Lancet* March:458–461, 1979.

Loggie JMH: Identification and management of juvenile hypertension. *Postgrad Med* 65:103–114, 1979.

Niarchos AP, Laragh JH: Hypertension in the elderly. I. Pathophysiology. *Mod Concepts Cardiovasc Dis* XLIX:43–48, 1980.

Niarchos AP, Laragh JH: Hypertension in the elderly. II. Diagnosis and treatment. *Mod Concepts Cardiovasc Dis* XLIX:49–54, 1980.

Task Force on Blood Pressure (National Heart, Lung, and Blood Institute): Report of the Task Force on Blood Pressure Control in Children. *Pediatrics* 59:797–820, 1977.

Chapter 22

Anderson RJ, Hart GR, Crumpler CP, Reed WG, Matthews CA: Oral clonidine loading in hypertensive urgencies. *JAMA* 246:848–850, 1981.

Gavras H, Brown WCB, Brown JJ, Lever AF, Linton AL, MacAdam RF, McNicol GP, Robertson JIS, Wardrop C: Microangiopathic hemolytic anemia and the development of the malignant phase of hypertension. *Circ Res* 28,29(Suppl II):II-127–II-141, 1971.

Grim CE: Management of malignant hypertension. *Front Med* 9:43–48, 1979.

Linton AL, Gavras H, Gleadle RI, Hutchison HE, Lawson DH, Lever AF, Macadam RF, McNicol GP, Robertson JIS: Microangiopathic haemolytic anaemia and the pathogenesis of malignant hypertension. *Lancet* June:1277–1282, 1969.

Luft FC, Bloch R, Szwed JJ, Grim CM, Grim CE: Minoxidil treatment of malignant hypertension. Recovery of renal function. *JAMA* 240:1985–1987, 1978.

Pickering G: Reversibility of malignant hypertension. Follow-up of three cases. *Lancet* February:413–418, 1971.

Raine AEG, Ledingham JGG: Clinical experience with captopril in the treatment of severe drug-resistant hypertension. *Am J Cardiol* 49:1475–1479, 1982.

Ram CVS: Captopril. *Arch Intern Med* 142:914–916, 1982.

Chapter 23

Armstrong JM, Blackwell GJ, Flower RJ, McGiff JC, Mullane KM, Vane JR: Genetic hypertension in rats is accompanied by a defect in renal prostaglandin catabolism. *Nature* 260:582–586, 1976.

Brody MJ: New developments in our knowledge of blood pressure regulation. *Fed Proc* 40:2257–2261, 1981.

Burris JF, Notargiacomo AV, Papademetriou V, Freis ED: Acute and short-term effects of a new calcium antagonist in hypertension. *Hypertenion* 4(suppl II)II-32–II-35, 1982.

Canessa M, Adragna N, Solomon HS, Connolly TM, Tosteson DC: Increased sodium–lithium countertransport in red cells of patients with essential hypertension. *N Engl J Med* 302:772–776, 1980.

Ferris TF: The kidney and hypertension. *Arch Intern Med* 142:1889–1895, 1982.

Garay RP, Elghozi J-L, Dagher G, Meyer P: Laboratory distinction between essential and secondary hypertension by measurement of erythrocyte cation fluxes. *N Engl J Med* 302:769–771, 1980.

Goodfriend TL: Receptors for angiotensins. In Genest J, Koiw E, Kuchel O (eds): *Hypertension.* New York, McGraw-Hill, 1977, pp 173–178.

Graham RM, Campbell WB: Speculative approaches in hypertension: Concepts and drugs of the future. *Fed Proc* 40:2291–2295, 1981.

Gruber KA, Whitaker JM, Buckalew VM Jr: Endogenous digitalis-like substance in plasma of volume-expanded dogs. *Nature* 287:743–745, 1980.

Haddy F, Pamnani M, Clough D: The sodium-potassium pump in volume expanded hypertension. *Clin Exp Hypertension* 1:295–336, 1978.

Henry PD: Comparative pharmacology of calcium antagonists: Nifedipine, verapamil and diltiazem. *Am J Cardiol* 46:1047–1058, 1980.

Kaplan HR, Smith RD: Antihypertensive drugs: Proposed sites and mechanisms of action. *Fed Proc* 40:2268–2274, 1981.

MacGregor GA, Smith SJ, Markandu ND, Banks RA, Sagnella GA: Moderate potassium supplementation in essential hypertension. *Lancet* September:567–570, 1982.

McCarron DA, Morris CD, Cole C: Dietary calcium in human hypertension. *Science* 217:267–269,

Michelakis AM, Mizukoshi H, Huang C, Murakami K, Inagami T: Further studies on the existence of a sensitizing factor to pressor agents in hypertension. *J Clin Endocrinol Metab* 41:90–96, 1975.

Muirheard EE, Byers LW, Desiderio DM, Brooks B, Brosius WM: Antihypertensive lipids from the kidney: Alkyl ether analogs of phosphatidylcholine. *Fed Proc* 40:2285–2290, 1981.

Poston L, Sewell RB, Wilkinson SP, Richardson PJ, Williams R, Clarkson EM, MacGregor GA, De Wardener HE: Evidence for a circulating sodium transport inhibitor in essential hypertension. *Br Med J* 282:847–849, 1981.

Index

D

R

S